Pı and *The*

"This motherfucker is of his squat."

—**Phil Letten**, *Vegan Bros*

"If you want to be a beast, then eat plant-based foods like the strongest beasts: gorillas, elephants, rhinos and other vegan powerhouses of the wild. In his new book, Daniel Austin shows you how. In addition to being an accomplished athlete, Daniel is incredibly passionate about helping others become their best version of themselves, having compassion for all, and I would totally take his advice."

—**Toni Okamoto**, *Plant Based on a Budget*

"The Way of The Vegan Meathead is an excellent read for anyone interested in veganism and lifting. Daniel writes from the heart about his personal experiences of being a 'Vegan Meathead' and shares his unique perspective. Daniel is the perfect example of what it means to be a compassionate man."

—**Natalie Matthews**, *Fit Vegan Chef* and NFF Bikini Pro

"Strong, funny, and hella tough, Daniel brings complete focus and dedication to everything he does, from hardcore to powerlifting, all the while keeping hard topics entertaining and interesting. He'll make you laugh while getting completely epic and yell 'Vegan Power!' as you lift more than you ever imagined."

—**Holly Noll** and **Ed Bauer**, *NewEthic Strength*

"Being a 'Vegan Meathead' myself, I feel a strong kinship with Daniel's writing. The tools he gives the reader of *The Way of The Vegan Meathead* are indispensable for creating a strong, healthy vegan body that can inspire others to follow the same path of ethical living."

—**Austin Barbisch**, author *Vegan Faster Stronger*

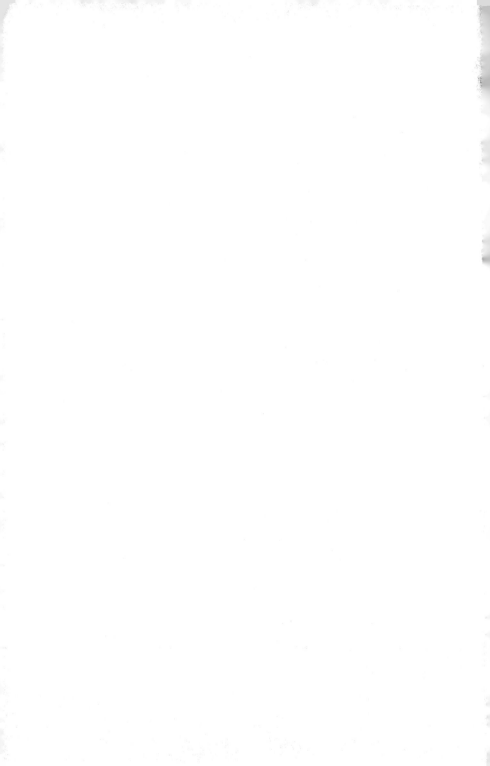

Disclaimer:

The advice given in this book is primarily based on personal experience, and is not intended to diagnose or treat any specific condition or illness. This is not a work of nutritional science, research, or peer-reviewed data. I am a vegan who lifts weights in my garage and eats more protein than most meat-eaters. This is simply what has worked for me over the course of years, and it very well may not work for you at all, but hey, it's worth a shot, right? And I'm only writing all of this since so many of you ask me for advice all the time. Try these recommendations at your own risk, and in the case of any complications, please seek help from a medical or nutritional expert. But whatever you do, do not give up on veganism, because that would be some weak ass shit. I am here to show you that when there is a will, there is indeed a way.

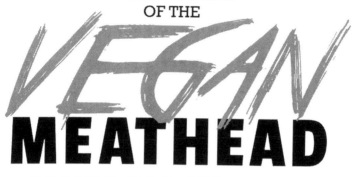

THE WAY OF THE VEGAN MEATHEAD

EATING FOR STRENGTH

DANIEL AUSTIN

First printed in the United States of America
by CreateSpace, 2018

Copyright © 2018 by Daniel Austin
Thank you for buying an authorized edition of this book.

Designed by Daniel Austin
Cover Art by Marc Strömberg
Logo Design by Garrett Huls

veg·an
ˈvēgən/
noun

a person who does not eat or use animal products

meat·head
ˈmētˌhed/
noun
informal

a muscular, but thick, person

veg·an meat·head
ˈvēgən/ mētˌhed/
noun, title of superiority

an apparent paradox which signifies the way of the future

FOR THE ANIMALS

CONTENTS

THE WAY OF THE VEGAN MEATHEAD — 1
MIGHT MAKES RIGHT — 4
EAT TO WIN — 7
High protein diets are harmful? — 7
Fake meat is fucking awesome — 14
Does not eating animals really give you a competitive advantage? — 18
Eating to win is NOT eating for fun (at least not always) — 21
If you're eating healthy foods, why do you still need supplements? — 23
Dude, why the fuck should we even listen to you anyway? — 24

FIBER: FRIEND AND FOE — 31

CARBOHYDRATES: CAN'T LIVE WITH 'EM, OR WITHOUT 'EM — 34
Preferred sources of complex carbs — 40
Preferred sources of simple carbs, glucose — 40

DON'T BE A FAT-OPHOBE — 41
Preferred sources of fat — 42

PROTEIN SOURCES: TO ANSWER YOUR FUCKING ETERNAL QUESTION — 43
Protein in natural foods — 44
Protein powders — 50
Meat analogs, a.k.a. fake meats — 60
Protein bars — 78

Not-enough-protein bars	83
Snacks	87

SUPPLEMENTS — 90
Non-optional supplements	91
Optional supplements	99
Things to not worry about	106

THE VEGAN MEATHEAD MEAL PLAN — 108
Lifting day meal plan	110
Regular off day / maintenance meal plan	117

SOME THOUGHTS ABOUT TRAINING — 122

GO FORTH NOW WITH A RIGHTEOUS MISSION — 128

ACKNOWLEDGEMENTS — 133

THE WAY OF THE VEGAN MEATHEAD

TO THIS DAY, despite the rising popularity of veganism, being vegan is still a relatively peculiar and socially taboo lifestyle. At best, according to various polls and estimates, only 3 to 5% of American adults are committed vegetarians, and of those pitifully low numbers only 1% or less claim to be vegan. That means if you're reading this you may be of a very ethical elite yet ostracized minority. Congratulations. Don't you just love explaining yourself awkwardly at every social gathering?

I don't know about you, but I know infinitely more people who have *tried* veganism than actual dedicated vegans. It seems that nearly everyone wants to try to align their sentiments of affinity and love for animals with their diet, but they try and fail because they genuinely have no clue how to balance their new fad diet to make themselves feel satiated, and then ultimately they resign themselves to the "fact" that eating the flesh and organs of tortured animals is just what people do. They blame the error of their ways on veganism itself, and then peddle the lie that it's just "human nature." Womp, womp.

Well, no, it's not universal human nature, as if there was such a thing, but it definitely is the nature of a passive nihilist to rely on such a weak fallacy for the rationalization of such preventable and immense suffering. If we're going to be perfectly honest with ourselves, truly, we must admit that this shitty, flimsy idea of "human nature" is a constantly changing thing, and therefore it does not exist. Imagine human nature one hundred years ago. It certainly wasn't human nature to fly in planes, watch sitcoms on television, listen to music on iPods, or jerk off to internet porn, but these days you can ask any guy, almost every single one alive currently, and they'll unanimously tell you, "Oh yeah, that's just what we do," as if things have always been this way...

The one universally good thing about the human species, and trust me when I say I am often hard-pressed to find anything good to say about our species, is that we do have the ability to become objectively aware of our behavior and our environment, and from there we also have the *potential* to *will* and *reason* calculated and thoughtful means of transforming our reality (extra emphasis on *potential*). We can do this for better or for worse, and we can do it every time we eat a meal in the privileged industrial world. A wise man once said that the "definition of *definition* is reinvention. To not be like your parents. To not be like your friends. To be yourself." This speaks to the idea of reinventing one's self *better*. Stronger. Wiser. That if we just accept what society and culture have prescribed for us to be then we are not being true to the idea of becoming our best possible self.

Another wise man once said "Man is something that should

be overcome," and that "What is great in Man is that he is a bridge and not a goal; what can be loved in man is that he is a *going-across* and a *down-going*."

See, the good news about so-called human nature is that it is *not* a static thing. This may bear some uncomfortable responsibility on us as individuals, but it does mean at any moment in our lives we can choose to not accept the way things are, should we be up to the task of putting in the work to change things. You and I stand on one side of an abyss, facing a greater state of ourselves on the other side. In between is all the suffering of the world, which includes the largest suffering class of all: the billions of animals who endure endlessly an existence of punishment, forced by human hands to wallow and languish in their own waste among their dead and diseased peers in feedlots, gestation crates, and battery cages; all for a diet that makes the privileged classes of our human peers sick, lethargic, and diseased while it deprives the lesser-privileged of the resources they need for survival; a diet that causes the remaining forests of the world to be clearcut for cattle grazing, which in turn accelerates global warming by depleting oxygen from our atmosphere, polluting our groundwater, and causing dead zones in our estuaries and oceans. We must go down and face these harsh and ugly realities, and we must emerge from them on the other side with the clarity and strength to do what benefits *everyone*.

That is *The Way of the Vegan Meathead*.

MIGHT MAKES RIGHT

I WENT VEGAN at the age of 22, going on 23 (back in 2005), and at that time I weighed about 135 pounds, 140 at best. I am a small guy by birthright: my mother isn't even 5 feet tall, and my father, the tallest in his family's history, is a mean 5 feet and 10 inches—not a small guy necessarily, but considering that both my grandfathers were 5'7" or so, and that all my uncles are anywhere between that and 5'9" at best, it is clear that the genetic odds of me being a naturally big, intimidating guy were never likely.

As you well know, the primary stereotypes vegans deal with on a daily basis—at least up until now, perhaps—is that of being weak and wimpy, and eating nothing but salad. I would be lying if I were to say that dealing with that stereotype has not influenced me to test the limits of my own strength—to push back against prevailing assumptions and prove people wrong for the sake of the animals. Granted, if you are just living as you do in order to prove other people wrong you're wasting your time, but some great motivation can come from being an underdog nonetheless. The process of becoming stronger has taught me many life lessons and boosted my capacity for self-discipline. It has also given me some advantages in the social sphere.

Fact: People generally react to you much differently when you emanate strength and confidence. People who come off as timid and weak are often overlooked or ignored by those who are larger or have more social currency. Those who look physically capable of overpowering you are naturally going to command more of your attention. I'm not saying it is fair, but it is the way it is.

I used to cower at the thought of getting in a fight or having to defend myself in a dire situation. Now, quite honestly, I'd welcome it. I know my strength, and there are times I'd just like to see what I can do with it if someone else should have a smart enough mouth. For better or for worse, that's the kind of testosterone boost eating tofu every day and squatting three times a week will give you. If anything, being vegan has only led me to approach life *more* aggressively, rather than the other way around.

Likewise, no one would have ever asked for my health or lifting advice as a scrawny 135 pound vegan, but now, as a competitive powerlifter thriving on a vegan diet, I get so overwhelmed with people asking for my help that I am writing this book. Even non-vegans (a.k.a. "soon-to-be-vegans") ask me for strength and health advice regularly. A little strength can go along way—both for personal wellness and self-esteem, as well as for helping the plight of our animal friends and the environment. Build yourself, and you will *make* people pay attention.

It is absolutely true that "might makes right." What you do with your might, though, makes all the difference in the world. You can use it to justify cruelty, or you can use it to overpower the forces of cruelty in the world. Let us choose to use our might for the latter.

In 2009 I went to work full-time for an animal rights organization. My work usually entailed outreach on college campuses or cultural events like concerts and festivals. My teams and I would generally try to engage people about the benefits of veganism or ask them to support specific animal rights campaigns. At the time, I was not yet into heavy weightlifting, and did not regularly enter the gym. At best I did calisthenics semi-regularly, and used a portable pull-up bar for pull-ups and push-ups when traveling. I ran some, too—nothing too specialized or goal-oriented. A few miles here or there. Nevertheless, that slight fitness edge over my coworkers who were less physically active often helped me reach more people to talk about issues, sign petitions, or take action against animal cruelty. People who would pass some of my coworkers by as they approached them often would not pass me by when I approached them. Sometimes assholes taunted them by eating meat in front of them, emphatically and on purpose. No one ever dared to do this to me. People often asked me if I was really vegan, and the frequency of that question only increased as I eventually got into heavy weight-lifting. Within a week of starting the job I was asked to manage traveling teams, as my bosses noticed that as soon I joined the team the behavior of the team changed, and they observed the responses of our audience in the field when I approached people there. It is undeniable: *might* makes a difference in getting people to listen, whether you like it or not. Every time someone out there encounters a strong vegan, they are forced to question their notion of what vegans are really like.

So let's get strong.

EAT TO WIN

IT IS OFTEN SAID among fitness fanatics, trainers, and bodybuilders that diet is 80% of your results. Of course, that is not a specific calculation, but the sentiment is correct: if you do not eat to adequately feed your muscles you will not get stronger, or you will only get as strong as your diet allows. Sleeping and exercise regimen also play a crucial role in fitness, but eating is huge. HUGE. And eating is likely the thing we all need the most discipline with.

So before we get started on how to eat properly to hone your potential strength, let's get some common misconceptions and disclaimers out of the way.

HIGH PROTEIN DIETS ARE HARMFUL?

Yes and no. High-protein animal-based diets have proven to be potentially harmful. Why? Mainly due to high cholesterol content (dietary cholesterol can *only* be found in animal-based foods) and lack of fiber (which slows the digestion process and allows for increased time to absorb fats and cholesterol from food). There is also the concern that elevated protein intake causes more calcium to be depleted from the bones to neutralize the acids used to break down proteins for digestion, increasing acidity in the body and stressing the kidneys, as well increasing the risk of osteoporosis (brittle bones) later in life.

Be rest assured though that even the experts, like T. Colin Campbell and Neal Barnard, have testified that plant-based protein sources have shown no evidence of causing the kinds of inflammation, acidity, kidney problems, or elevated cholesterol levels that are associated with animal-based protein sources. Even so, these same doctors try to market plant-based diets which are low in protein. While I sympathize with the efforts of these experts—and the Forks Over Knives/ What the Health movement in general—to divorce the general population from the dogma that protein is the most important element of diet to consider, I must dissent that protein is vital to strength athletes—especially powerlifters, bodybuilders, and strongmen. Sure, protein is of virtual non-importance to the average sedentary American, as whole plant foods will provide more than enough of a variety of amino acids to meet basic protein requirements for people who do not exert themselves at an elite level, but we must recognize that the whole food, low protein diet that Forks Over Knives and its advocates recommend is for one kind of person—a normal person who doesn't engage in extreme weight-bearing exercise. The diet I am promoting in this book is for another kind of person—a *Vegan Beast*. I suppose if you have no interest in becoming a Vegan Beast you can just stop reading now and go back to watching Netflix while munching on a bowl of some carb-heavy, low-protein bullshit snack food like chips or whatever typical useless garbage you people like to eat.

And sure, consuming an abundant amount of protein is of much less importance to endurance athletes like runners, fighters, cyclists or swimmers, but for athletes who need muscles that can move weights that are many times more than their own bodyweight, increased protein consumption is necessary. It is all relative to your fitness goals.

For example, champion UFC fighter (and vegan), Mack Danzig showed that his diet rarely included more than 80g of protein per day. A lot of his protein sources are fully natural whole foods like beans and chickpeas, and tofu or tempeh. He relied very little on supplements and fake meats. Champion ultra-marathoner and Iron Man, Brendan Brazier (creator of Vega supplements), stated that he rarely eats more than 60g of protein a day, especially when competing. He even eschews the consumption of soy, citing it as "inflammatory." From what I have seen in online interviews with him, the man seems to live on Vega and salad pretty much—and that is okay because his goals require him to eat much differently than I, or any other strength athlete may be required to do, despite him being a very tall man who likely weighs about the same or less than me (a notably short man). His stance, and he's right, is that for endurance athletes, increased muscle mass is a detractor of performance. It entails more mass that the athlete has to move repetitively, and doing so will wear the athlete out sooner than his competitors who are lighter in frame and fill.

For Brendan Brazier and Scott Jurek (vegan, champion long distance runner), and any of these types of athletes who depend on slow-twitch muscle performance for their endurance, less protein is needed in their diet. More protein can equate to more body mass (when coupled with a correct training regimen), and that is just not practical for someone who wants to be really fast at a repetitive thing like running or cycling. And likewise, for a cage fighter like Mack Danzig, too much mass can mean throwing a slower punch, even though it may be a stronger punch, or perhaps not being able to throw as many fast punches, whereas a powerlifter is relying on fast-twitch muscle performance for maximal strength output in very short bursts that he will usually not have to repeat more than a small number of times in training, and not even more than once in competition. Proper conditioning for a powerlifter requires virtually no aerobic capacity, at least not nearly the aerobic capacity comparable to a marathoner or fighter.

As you can see, the discussion about endurance sports and strength sports is generally a discussion about two different types of strength, which call for different types of diet planning. As a general rule, the more mobile and cardio-intensive your fitness goals are, the less important a steady flow of protein will be in your daily meal plan. And vice versa, the more you are aiming for short displays of maximal strength which create multitudes of micro-tears through a variety of muscle groups, the more you will need to focus on upping your protein intake.

To be very clear, *again*, this book is for those looking to build muscle mass and increase strength. I have no adequate experience to give tips to anyone about being a good fighter or endurance athlete. I ceased to be personally interested in that kind of performance quite a while ago, once I realized that to be exceptionally good at strength sports it would require that I cease to be good at other sports which require more endurance. That's not a knock on endurance sports. It's just a matter of my own preference.

Moreover, this book is also for those who want to learn to build strength while also managing weight or losing weight. My interest in competitive powerlifting has taught me that to be competitive in any given weight class, one must eat appropriate proportions of calories and macronutrients to maintain, add, or cut weight as needed. For most people, bulking is no problem, so much of what I will divulge going forward will be about weight maintenance and losing weight while not losing strength (as that is the trick which requires the most dietary discipline).

Now, back to why diets high in plant-based protein are not problematic the way diets high in animal-based protein are. As everyone knows, or should know, there is no cholesterol in plant-based food, only in animal-based food, so we understand that plant proteins are heart-healthy in the capacity that they are associated with a much lower risk of clogging arteries or developing symptoms of heart disease. Generally speaking, there is no cause for concern about high cholesterol or clogged arteries with a vegan diet.

However, just so that I am being perfectly fair, some people have naturally higher cholesterol due to genetic conditions, even vegans. I have met vegans who have confided this information about themselves to me. It is not impossible to have high cholesterol as a vegan, and certainly eating high quantities of oils and processed sugars, no matter whether you eat animal flesh, bodily secretions or not, *can potentially* complicate hereditary cholesterol-related issues by increasing arterial inflammation. Statistically though, these conditions among vegans are undeniably less common by vast numbers, and are more of an exception to the general rule that eating no dietary cholesterol usually helps maintain healthy endogenic cholesterol levels than anything else. If you get online and search for studies comparing total cholesterol levels between vegans, vegetarians, and omnivores, you will routinely find that the results show vegans on average maintain lower total cholesterol than omnivores, often by 30-50 points in men, and 20-30 points in women, and vegetarians are usually in the middle. See for yourself.

If you are a vegan with genetic issues related to cholesterol, do please tread carefully with what I propose in this book. It is possible that a low oil, low fat diet will be more beneficial for you, and I do recommend seeking professional counsel if you are one of those rare cases. In most cases with most people though, these concerns are going to be irrelevant. Nevertheless, it is wise to track your own cholesterol two to three times a year to see how you are holding up, whether you decide to follow The Way of The Vegan Meathead or not.

Furthermore, we understand that plant-based food is typically lower in saturated fat, as well as higher in fiber, so generally speaking, plant foods that move through our digestive tract are generally there for less time, meaning there is usually less time for fat absorption. Though I will describe the drawbacks of higher fiber intake for vegans seeking to build muscle mass in a bit, do note that finding a healthy balance between fiber, protein, fat, and carbohydrate intake is key to succeeding as a vegan strength athlete. No matter how you slice the bread, fiber is essential, and without it you are going to degrade the quality of your life in the long run. It promotes the flourishing of healthy gut bacteria which can help you break down proteins for absorption even though excessive amounts of protein can reduce the amount of time you have to absorb protein. Likewise fiber can attach itself to bile generated from cholesterol excreted by your liver to help flush it out your colon. In other words, fiber is really good for your long term health. These kinds of benefits are not typically associated with low fiber, animal based diets, and as you will see in my meal plan later on, the diet I am promoting here is still adequate for meeting daily fiber intake recommendations according to leading nutrition experts and organizations, yet it is lower in fiber compared to most variations of a vegan diet.

Ah, yes, but what about stress on the kidneys? More protein consumption means more work for the kidneys to do, and eating excessive amounts of plant protein, be it soy or other, still means more work for the kidneys just the same…right?

Apparently NO according to Michael Greger, M.D. Meat, dairy, and egg consumption reportedly causes "hyperfiltration" and "protein leakage" in the kidneys, and the overall taxation of the kidneys by an animal-centric diet on a daily basis is compared to running a car's engine into the red at every meal. Over time, the build-up of ammonia and renal acid leads to gout, kidney stones, and even kidney failure. Luckily, prolonged consumption of plant protein, even protein-isolates and elevated plant protein intake has yet to illustrate evidence of spiking kidney function at all in numerous studies. On average, when processing plant protein, a healthy human kidney continues humming while doing business as usual.

This doesn't mean you shouldn't be drinking water all the time. *Of course* you should be drinking water all the time. Staying hydrated and then some is the best thing you can do for your kidneys and *every cell in your body*, no matter what, whether you eat a high protein plant-protein diet or not. Just because plant protein is proven to be easier on your kidneys, staying hydrated is always top priority.

FAKE MEAT IS FUCKING AWESOME

Since we've gotten it out of the way that plant protein is no problem for your kidneys, and that the plant protein bogeyman doesn't exist, let's talk about fake meat and why you *should* eat it. Some decry, like my mother, the Forks Over Knives crowd, and holistic foodies in general, that fake meat is "not natural!" It's "high in sodium!" It's not "whole food!" being that much of is based of wheat gluten or soy protein isolate. "IT'S PROCESSED, OMG!" Protein powder "isn't food at all!" Likewise they claim supplements are unnecessary, because "whole foods can give you all you need!" "All that soy (or gluten) can't be good for you!"

Okay, people, I recognize your concerns, but can you show me another vegan in the 165 pound open raw weight class whose Big 3 lifts amount to well over 7x their bodyweight, or have a Wilks score of 400? To be fair, I know of a few vegan lifters who are on this level, but my deadlift is currently triple my bodyweight, and my most recent total in competition is hovering around 1,200 pounds. Sure, maybe there are other vegans at my level of strength out there (I do know a few), but I guarantee you they are eating roughly as much protein as I am, and getting that much per day is much harder—and less enjoyable—without fake meat. Sure, Torre Washington, a.k.a. "The Vegan Dread" exists, and he is a professional bodybuilder who does zero supplementation (as is evidenced by his website and videos on his YouTube channel), but he is an anomaly, and even so he definitely eats fake meat. Regardless, if there is going to be a shift away from high protein consumption in strength and physique sports, it is going to come as more and more champions in the sport drift away from it by proving that they can win without it. That is going to be a process—if it ever happens—which occurs over time. In the meantime, however, I can tell you my bloodwork shows that I am perfectly healthy as I continue to eat 200+ grams of protein per day, and have been doing so for years.

I can also tell you that many of the vegan bodybuilders I have come to know are doing higher carb diets than I do, but they also emphasize protein intake—regularly consuming more than 200g most days of the week. Granted, many of them also consume much higher calories than I do, and most of them are carbohydrate based, which comes with more fiber intake as well. Personally, I prefer to consume less calories and rely a bit more on fat calories for energy, as fat comes with no fiber attached, which can potentially help slow digestion in order to create more time to absorb amino acids in order to better rebuild muscle (another thing to consider is that bodybuilders focus on hypertrophy—more reps at lighter weight—than powerlifters—who focus on maximal strength, and therefore bodybuilders and physique competitors typically create less micro-tears in muscle fiber because they do not often work with loads above 85% of their one-rep max, and with that in mind, elevated protein intake may also be slightly less important for bodybuilders than powerlifters).

In regard to soy and gluten being bad for you, since there is so much hearsay and hysteria about soy and gluten these days, the truth is that if you don't have an actual diagnosable allergy or intolerance to them, there is no issue with eating them. Some people *do* have those adverse reactions to soy or gluten, and that's definitely a real thing for some people, but it is really *not* a real thing for most people. I wouldn't call gluten a superfood by any means—it is definitely super tasty and filling—but soy, without a doubt, is high in protein, iron, calcium, folic acid, and contains a significant level of omega-3 fatty acids. Organic soy won't make you grow manboobs or disrupt your testosterone production. The only kind of soy in question which may potentially contribute to that is GMO soy which is fed almost exclusively to livestock (and guess which kind of people eat that kind of soy, even if only indirectly), and even then you'd need to eat it by the truckload like a forlorn cow trapped on a feedlot to disrupt your hormones, as it is likely that a little GMO here or there isn't going to noticeably affect your hormone levels. Basically, people who say soy increases estrogen deserve to get punched in the fucking face. I guess all the meat-eaters who have placed lower than me at powerlifting meets must eat more soy than me.

Why fake meat then, you ask? One reason why is that some fake meats are relatively high in protein while being low in carbs and fat. If you are trying to build muscle and maintain or lose weight that is important to consider. You can make fake meat the centerpiece of your meals, and it will help you stay full and content with the flavor of your meals.

But beware, *not all fake meats are created equally*. Sadly, it's true, and you will see later in the Vegan Meathead meal plan that I only recommend specific fake meats, and that is for good reason. Tofu on its own is also great, as it is are relatively low carb, but tempeh—due to its higher carb content—is not a regular choice of mine, as much as it is a healthy fermented food, and tasty too. There are also certain brands of fake meat that I love the taste of, but they sometimes have more carbs than protein, and that is just not going to cut it if I have bodyweight goals to make for competition, or to just consistently increase strength without gaining bodyfat.

Oh, but fake meats have a lot of sodium, and that makes

you retain water, and that can't be good for cutting weight? Guess what else has a lot of sodium. Milk, cheese, deli meats, hot dogs, sausages, pretty much any kind of fried or battered version of a meat product you can think of, and just about anything you buy that is canned or packaged. So before you let anyone else criticize you for eating protein sources that are sometimes high in sodium, make sure motherfuckers check themselves about what they eat, too. Perhaps fake meats are not perfect foods. I would never claim that they are. Yes, they typically have relatively high sodium content, but unless you develop the symptoms of edema (swelling caused by water retention, often in the extremities and face), or extreme thirst, odds are your sodium levels are fine. And to be sure, sodium is an electrolyte which helps regulate muscle function. Your body actually *needs* sodium. It is only harmful in regular large quantities and most often only affects older people and people who are immobile or do not exercise much. If you're a lifter or an athlete of some kind, then you run a very low risk of being affected by sodium from eating fake meats. To this day, I have yet to meet a vegan with a sodium-induced problem, but to be safe, I also recommend eating lots of natural foods, steamed or in their natural state, to counter the amount of sodium you may be eating from fake meat.

Something else to consider is that the daily recommended intake for sodium is 2300mg per day or less, and even that is highly contested among researchers. Some would say that 2000-3500mg is a perfectly acceptable intake range for an overall healthy adult. On the other hand, eating too little sodium can be dangerous, and it is most often the raw foodists and obsessive macrobiotic adherents who run the risk of eating too little sodium.

As you will see, I rarely eat fake meats by themselves, and

include vegetables in my diet most times I eat. Fake meats are important to The Way of the Vegan Meathead, but are not The Way themselves.

DOES NOT EATING ANIMALS REALLY GIVE YOU A COMPETITIVE ADVANTAGE?

Some say yes. Some say no. I say it depends on what you mean by "advantage." If you are talking about overall health and longevity, I would say veganism, even the Vegan Meathead style of veganism presented in this book, is likely to give you an advantage in life, in the long-term, via decreased risk of the major killers in western society (heart disease, colon cancer, prostate cancer, diabetes, etc.), as well as decreasing your likelihood for obesity, impotence, Alzheimer's, and other conditions which can greatly decrease your quality of life. It is well documented that a balanced vegan diet is a great way to combat and alleviate all of those problems and more, but to say it gives you a competitive advantage in sport may be a leap too far. Besides, remember: we are vegans because it is the right thing to do; a way to improve humanity, care for animals, and the environment that sustains us.

I recall Carl Lewis' recount of his Olympic running team. He said that many of the athletes he trained with often had the worst diets imaginable. He said that once he became a vegetarian and then a vegan, he began winning more, and then his peers began to take note and follow his example for a while, but he also said he was still in a very competitive field and of course did not always win despite his improved diet. It is important to consider that despite your best efforts to eat an optimal diet, there will always be assholes who are more genetically advantaged than you. You know them, those pricks who eat garbage and pastries every day, but still looked ripped and run laps around the rest of us. It's just a fact of life. It doesn't mean, however, that you should give up on an ethically superior diet, because *that* would show weak character.

Someone like Michael Phelps burns so many calories swimming for hours per day that it makes almost no difference what he eats, at least in regards to short term effects on performance. The penultimate factor of being able to fuel one's body adequately for sport is apparently not what kind of calories one gets, but the sheer fact of whether they get enough calories to begin with (and that, my friends, is one major crux of the problem for so many who flirt with veganism since plant-based foods are usually less calorically dense than animal-based shit). I would also say it depends on which kind of sport we're talking about. We are seeing a boom in boxers and fighters adopting (at least mostly) vegan eating plans to accommodate their training regimens (Nate Diaz, Mack Danzig, Jake Shields, Tim Bradley to name a few), as well as football players (David Carter, Griff Whalen), and while some of them are leading their pack, some of them are not. There are so many factors involved in regard to what makes one a superior athlete in his or her sport that I cannot in good conscience tell you that simply being vegan will give you Vegan Power to help you demolish your competition. You have to learn how to cultivate your own Vegan Power. Seriously, I mean that. It is going to be a process that requires discipline and dedication. More important than what you stand to lose or gain by becoming vegan, or competing as a vegan athlete, is the ethical stance that killing and eating animals is unjust because it is no longer necessary for the advancement and survival of our species.

Whether veganism gives you an advantage or not, it all boils down to the big question: *How badly do you want to be strong as a vegan?* Ultimately it is up to you to redefine and reinvent yourself in your own vision. Do you hunger for the new you and a new world? And are you going to do what it takes to make yourself live up to your own ideals? Are you going to do what it takes to prove that veganism really is the future? Evolution doesn't happen when species sit around getting their asses kicked by circumstances until they are buried by extinction. Circumstances will beat you down, but growth, change, and transformation only occur when we rise up and *will* ourselves to the next step.

So let that be your advantage: you're here to represent something bigger than yourself and change the world, and currently the odds are very much against you. Let that resistance fuel you. We're going to have to do some serious work to change people's understanding of diet and health, and how it all relates to animals, the planet, and each other. When veganism is universally known as the antonym for feebleness, we're going to be so much closer to the compassionate and just world we want to live in. At the very least, people are going to think twice about arguing with us.

EATING TO WIN IS NOT EATING FOR FUN (AT LEAST NOT ALWAYS)

I love my diet. I don't mean this lightly at all: I enjoy eating more as a vegan than when I wasn't yet vegan. The reason for this revelation is that going vegan forced me out of the comfort zone I lived in as a teenager and young adult—the comfort zone of eating processed shit and fast food all the time. Pizza, fast food burgers, frozen burritos covered in cheese, fish sticks, boxed macaroni, sugary cereals, Ramen noodles, Hot Pockets, Little Debbie snacks, and fruit roll-ups, chicken fingers. It is a true miracle I didn't sentence myself to long term metabolic damage or diabetes with the kind of garbage I was eating when left to my own devices as a kid. I suppose that's a true testament to the resilience of the evolution of the human body. I continued to eat much of the same kinds of garbage through my teenage years, even when I became a pescetarian at 15. But once I went vegan there were very few of the kinds of mock alternatives to those kinds of foods on the market at the time. I had to learn about falafel, curry, tempeh, Ethiopian lentils, chana masala, and so much more. There was a whole world of flavor out there that I was not eating my whole life prior simply because I had been living in the American fast food-pizza-hamburger-sugary snack bubble.

Nevertheless, I do not intend to say that I eat a great variety of international cuisine all the time. Truthfully speaking, I do not. Doing so is not required to achieve the goals I have set for myself, and furthermore, eating out at restaurants on a regular basis is not only expensive, but it is the worst way to know how many calories you are eating, let alone how many fat calories or grams of carbs you are eating. According to

Michael Pollan (who is, in my estimation, a sometimes fair omnivore), all the populations of people throughout the world who have the healthiest body mass indexes are the people who make their own food the most (Note: I am not a fan of body mass indexing, as a muscular powerlifter, my weight is almost alarmingly high for my height, which is of course bullshit. I only refer to BMI as a very general, non-specific indicator of overall health that some people seem to care about.) The theory is that if you can see how much salt, or butter (errr Earth Balance), or sugar, or oil you are putting into a pot, the more likely you are to have reservations about using higher quantities of those kinds of calorie-dense substances, whereas when you go out to eat in a restaurant, keeping tabs on those quantities is virtually impossible. Rest assured though that the food you eat in a restaurant tastes as incredible as it perhaps does because the cook likely put more of those forbidden magic ingredients in your dish to keep you hooked on the flavor and coming back for more. It's good for business, sure, but maybe not for your fitness goals.

Which brings us to a very important point: How *good* food tastes has nothing to do with whether you should be eating it or not. In fact, the better it tastes the more likely it is that you should not eat it, or at least eat it less often. You may cringe at the thought of eating plain Tofurky sausage with a cup of steamed broccoli twice each afternoon, but take some comfort in knowing that you will be getting what you *need* from it, and that is the bottom line. It may not seem so appealing to eat meals that are 300 calories or less several times a day, but again—it is all about getting what you need and nothing more. Likewise, the thought of eating no sweets, or fruit, or a very limited amount of carbs (which come primarily from green vegetables) for nearly all your daylight hours may seem like torture, but I tell you it's probably what you *need*. So get used to satisfying your needs and stopping there. Eating to meet your needs is most often not going to taste as decadent as you'd like, but that is okay.

IF YOU'RE EATING HEALTHY FOODS, WHY DO YOU STILL NEED SUPPLEMENTS?

The fact of the matter is that when you put your body through the wringer for a long time, over and over again, like someone who steadily trains for strength gains, then food alone is probably not going to help you absorb every kind of nutrient you need to absorb to stay in the best possible shape—not without adding more calories. This is especially true if you have to gain strength yet stay under a certain weight limit like competitive powerlifters or olympic weightlifters must do. If you're the kind of otherwise vain person who just wants to burn fat and maintain mass, or perhaps even get stronger while losing weight, then this would also apply to you.

For example, each gram of fat you eat has about 9 calories. That's a lot of energy compared to carbs or protein (which on average contain about 4 calories per gram), and generally speaking, with the exception of when the body reaches ketosis, adding fat calories to your diet is going to make you store more fat, gain weight and mass that will have no practical use for your goal of gaining strength, simply because fat contains more than double the calories of either protein or carbohydrates.

Take for example Omega-3 fatty acid. Whether vegan or

not, the food-based sources of Omega-3 are attached to many calorically-dense fatty calories. For soon-to-be vegans, prime sources are fish oil, fish flesh, and eggs. For vegans, prime sources are walnuts, and various forms of seeds like chia, flax, and hemp—all of which are relatively high calorie and ought to be eaten in small portions when one needs to keep weight and body fat goals in mind. Omega-3 is important for brain function and forming anti-inflammatory compounds (which are of dire importance for lifters of heavy-ass weight), so we simply cannot skimp on it. Since we can't reasonably eat nuts and oils all day without exceeding our caloric limits for weight maintenance, taking low calorie gelatinless capsules of Omega 3 can be vital to helping you achieve your beastly goals.

Another example is taking Calcium-Magnesium-Zinc. Sure, if you're regularly eating broccoli, leafy greens, tofu, beans and other Calcium and Magnesium rich plant foods (of which there are a plethora), you may be wondering why someone ought to take a supplement for such minerals. There are a couple reasons for this. One is that when you put your central nervous system, joints, ligaments, and muscles under extreme stress consistently for a long time you accumulate higher than normal levels of inflammation, and from there you may risk needing more of certain minerals and nutrients to reduce that inflammation (As you can see here, the common pattern is one that minimizes caloric intake while achieving a reduction of inflammation). One symptom of lacking Magnesium is muscle twitching, which I have experienced, but only after many years of lifting. Magnesium is critical for muscle contraction, nerve transmission, and cell formation. If you aren't getting enough Magnesium, your most strained muscles may twitch. While it's not painful, it is a subtle signal of insufficient mineral levels in your blood. I never experienced said muscle twitching when I was a vegan who wasn't lifting heavy, but after years of lifting heavy I was alarmed by when I first experienced some twitching and have found that a Calcium-Magnesium-Zinc pill once or twice on a daily basis helps to calm it, and it is an adequate source that doesn't require me to eat more calories. Calcium also helps neutralize inflammation in the body and can potentially help burn fat, so that is a bonus.

To be clear, I still eat as many natural sources of these minerals as I can. Supplementation is never an excuse to forego getting nutrients and minerals from more natural sources, which are primarily vegetables. The sooner you understand that there is no way around eating vegetables every damn day, the better. Only five-year-olds try to avoid eating vegetables. Some of you are going to have to grow up if you want to achieve Vegan Power.

I will talk more about supplements later on in this book, and go into greater detail about which supplements I recommend, at which times, and why.

DUDE, WHY THE FUCK SHOULD WE EVEN LISTEN TO YOU ANYWAY?

Fair question. I encourage you to be skeptical of me, and of anyone promoting dietary solutions. There are a million reports and perspectives about what kind of diet works best. So much so, that it is truly impossible to say there is one, or are even a few superior diets out there. The truth is that there are many ways to achieve your diet and fitness goals, and furthermore, not all of them will work for everyone, but many of them will work for lot of people if they have enough discipline to follow a meal and exercise plan.

For example, high-carb veganism is definitely having a moment right now, especially in the bodybuilding sector, but I can tell you that when I explored a high carb approach, or at the very least, when I did not limit my carbs, I got fatter, and at a point I wasn't getting stronger either—not at a proportion that justified all the carbs I was eating. I won't deny it works for some people, but doing the high carb thing entails a ton of fiber, and there are many drawbacks to shitting four to seven times a day (of which I will spare explaining to you in detail), but I am sure you can adequately employ your imagination about that.

As for my credentials, they are really not very impressive on an academic level. I was a certified personal trainer for a bit, but didn't enjoy it much for a wide variety of reasons (mostly because it was like babysitting), and I hated paying and repaying for certifications. I learned the most as a personal trainer by mingling and networking with other trainers about what works and what doesn't for different types of people. Wisdom comes from experience, not textbooks. Sometimes anyway.

A lot of what training certification textbooks teach you is proper exercise form based on general physiology for you to teach to weak people so that they don't get injured and you don't get your ass sued. The kind of form strength athletes learn to improve their squat, deadlift, or bench often defies the safe techniques taught in personal training courses.

Examples: rounding shoulders when necessary on heavy deadlifts, looking down when deadlifting or squatting, arching back as much as possible to decrease range of motion and engage lats on a bench press, or squatting below parallel. Those are just a few examples of some key things to learn for powerlifting technique, but for an average person, or an older, previously injured person, they could spell disaster.

Likewise, pilates balls, BOSU balls, machines, abdominal isolation exercises, or cardio in general, are all pretty much fucking useless to a strength athlete. I learned all that the hard way by becoming a strength athlete over the course of years of trial and error in regard to diet and training. So how nice it is that you get to simply read this book and learn the wisdom I gained from years of sucking at vegan fitness? It was a long road to figure out how to become decent at my shit. I hope yours is much shorter.

Regarding my nutritional credentials, I assure you I have even less than my training credentials. In fact I have none, and most of my knowledge about vegan strength nutrition has come from reading books and the internet (LOL!), and then trying to incorporate various macronutrient balances and supplemental approaches to my own diet, and again, learning what works for me and what doesn't through trial and error. In the end, it's the results that matter, right? Plus, in my defense, at least I can say I have been vegan for twelve years, a competitive vegan athlete for more than two and a half, and in all that time I have only gotten healthier and stronger. In fact, by the eating methods I have devised, along with ever-evolving training methods, I have been able to put 200 pounds on my total powerlifting score while gaining zero bodyweight. That's ultimately what counts, and it's why people ask my advice all the time.

On top of that, I've at least taken the consideration to hire a registered dietitian to review this book for me and help me explain my nutritional approach in the least inaccurate ways possible. Sounds promising, huh? After reviewing this whole book for me, I asked her "On a scale of one to ten, how problematic is this diet I am promoting?" Her response: Only "a five or a six!" HA! To be fair, she also declared the caveat that that was only in her educated opinion, that she sees that what I do on a daily basis obviously works for me, that my methods thus far have had no obvious side-effects for me, and being that so much is still unaccounted for in the world of nutritional science, especially in regard to the individual differences between each of us, she can't ultimately deem The Way of The Vegan Meathead as unhealthy or unethical (so long as I advise readers to proceed according to my advice with caution, which I of course always will).

If nothing else, I can tell you this: I started competing in powerlifting in 2015, at the age of 32 (kind of late in the game, to be honest). In late 2014 I started eating more or less by the meal plan I divulge to you toward the end of this book in order to prepare to make weight for my first meet, because I realized that in order for my numbers to even be semi-competitive, I needed to get into a lighter weightclass. I also quit doing cardio then to focus on utilizing all my calories for strength gains and max lifts instead of warm-up bullshit. My strategy proved to be successful, and I made weight for the 165 pound/75kg weightclass in June 2015.

In two and a half years of eating this way I've dropped bodyfat percentage by about 6%, and reached a point of balance for my body where I now hover around 12% bodyfat most of the time, and weigh more than 20 pounds less than when I started eating this way and training only for strength. I am also much stronger than when I was not eating this way and training only for strength. I am now strong enough to compete on a national level in both the United States Powerlifting Association (USPA) and the USA Powerlifting (USAPL) organization, which is also part of the International Powerlifting Federation (IPF), the leading powerlifting organization in the world. My deadlift qualifies as a Master level lift according to USPA's qualification standards, and I am quickly approaching an Elite level for my weightclass, of which there is only one higher level (International Elite). It is fair to say I am not the strongest guy around, but for a vegan in a sport dominated exponentially by non-vegans (a.k.a. soon-to-be-vegans), I'm doing more than alright, as I have won meets, placed in the top three in many, and I am always working on the means to become better. I've also done all this nearly injury-free and without a coach, which is practically unheard of and would likely be impossible without a solid diet to back it up. In the end, results are all that matter.

One last thing about diet: Yes, there are many roads to the same destination, and though I promote a lower carb vegan diet than a lot of vegan athletes otherwise do, I have my reasons for it, and I will attempt to make them all as clear to you in this book as I can. By no means do I think my way is the only way to achieve your goals, but my methods work for me, and I can only tell you my story and my methods as I know them. The Way of The Vegan Meathead is one way to build strength. It is not the way for everyone.

The biggest factor of maintaining or losing bodyfat is undoubtedly training while sticking to a slight caloric deficit with your eating habits. I have done this for many years, and I have seen firsthand that you can lose fat and gain strength simultaneously if you do it all at the proper rate. This means no drastic weight-cuts. Instead of drastic cuts, you engage in a slow, sustainable process of leaning out over a longer period of time until you figure out your natural boundaries for losing, maintaining, and gaining both bodyweight and strength. If your protein intake is high enough you can maintain and even build muscle while losing fat and bodyweight. Perhaps you can do this while eating higher quantities of carbs—as long as you maintain a slight caloric deficit, and perhaps you can do it eating higher quantities of fat calories (as I do), but again it still boils down to maintaining a slight caloric deficit. I find relying on fat to be more advantageous because more fat equates to less fiber, and that potentially slows digestion a bit to give you more time to absorb proteins and make use of them, as I have said before, and will say again many times in this book.

But by all means, if it doesn't work for you, then fuck it. Try something else. There is nothing EVER that is bound to work for everyone. I'd be lying if I guaranteed you anything.

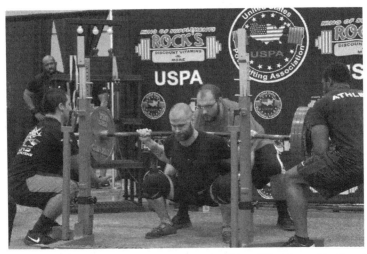

Squatting deep is also an important part of The Way of The Vegan Meathead. Squat deep or fuck off. (Photo: Crystal Moulton)

FIBER: FRIEND *AND* FOE

AN UNCOMFORTABLE overlying issue that a lot of vegans don't want to talk about is *fiber*. Yep, fiber. Fiber is a tricky thing. It's essential to colorectal and digestive health, but at this same time, since fiber is either indigestible (insoluble fiber) or helps with the gradual conversion of food into stored energy (soluble fiber), it causes things to move through our bodies faster than they otherwise would if they weren't attached to fiber. In that way fiber is much like a broom used for tidying the house, sweeping all the junk out the backdoor. One reason meat-eaters are statistically plagued by colon cancer, irritable bowel syndrome, and higher bodyweight (the list goes on…) is because animal products contain no fiber, and therefore the things they often eat sit in their bodies much longer, allowing more time for absorption of fats, carcinogenic compounds, and dietary cholesterol. There is also much evidence about the many ways fiber enriches the microbiome in our guts, which aids in building our immune system.

Likewise, one reason vegans sometimes find it hard to gain weight or muscle mass is because our diets are made up almost entirely of fiber-rich foods that are less calorically-dense than animal-based foods to begin with. While that means our intestines may store less waste than omnivores, it also means we have less time to absorb things that help us gain strength, like the amino acids that are the building blocks of proteins which help repair and rebuild muscles after a hard workout.

The Way of The Vegan Meathead is, in part, the method of finding a balance between natural healthy plant foods, and supplementation to optimize nutrient and amino acid absorption to gain strength. One reason I am so adamant about consuming more protein, whether through protein-dense foods, or be it through supplementation, is that fiber can prevent us from utilizing a significant portion of the protein we consume. Fiber reduces the *bio-availability* of proteins in our body. Taking supplements is just one means of trouble-shooting natural roadblocks to gaining strength. Not only this, but fiber is very filling, so it can make you feel full sooner, and that feeling of fullness can sometimes prevent you from eating enough calories or grams of protein to make the gains you are seeking.

Fiber is actually a lot like cardio. Pesky cardio. It's great for your heart's health, but it really can work steadfastly against making strength gains. Over the years, I've proudly quit doing cardio altogether, yet found a dietary way to limit my body fat percentage (I've even decreased body fat without cardio), and it just so happens that the dietary means I have primarily been implemented by increasing the amount of foods I eat that lack fiber, like fats and oils, simple carbohydrates (which are timed specifically for optimal effect), and high protein consumption. See, the thing about veganism is that it can easily entail a high fiber diet even when you try to limit the fiber in it. You will see this quantified in the chart of the meal plan later on.

The recommended daily intake for a normal adult male is 38g of fiber per day, and my take on low-fiber veganism still gets you close enough to that 38g recommendation to be no cause for worry. Comparatively, American men eat a wimpy average of 18g of fiber a day. The potential consequences of regularly eating that little fiber begin with constipation, diarrhea, diverticulitis, and other more threatening conditions that plague the colon, like cancer. Consistently not eating enough fiber is like taking your digestive system out back and beating the shit out of it.

Primarily, the most abundant sources of fiber are going to come from fruits, vegetables, and grains—those fecund sources of complex carbohydrates which are all great in their own right, but like I said before, sometimes they sweep things through your guts so fast you don't get time to absorb all the amino acids you need to be absorbing to reach your next level of Vegan Power. Thus we must learn when to eat fiber-rich foods and when not to, which brings us to the ever-controversial: *Carbohydrates*.

CARBOHYDRATES: CAN'T LIVE WITH 'EM, OR WITHOUT 'EM

I'M NOT HERE to tell you carbohydrates will make you fat. Nor am I here to tell you carbohydrates are the key to unlocking your greatest potential. Some people say you don't need them, yet they are nearly impossible to avoid. But to be fair, those people who say you don't need them likely get all their vitamins from supplements, and I abide by the rule that the best way to get vitamins is not from supplements. We supplement simply because when we push our bodies to their limits we need extra vitamins.

One thing that is for certain is that your main load of daily carbohydrates ought to be complex carbohydrates from vegetables. Fuck oatmeal, fuck brown rice, or quinoa. Just eat vegetables. Anecdotally speaking, regularly eating rice and cereals *does* make me get fat, and because of how much fiber they have I have to go to the bathroom way too often. For the most part rice, cereals, and noodles are just filler in your meals. They are not the best tasting parts of your meals, and they certainly are not the most protein or nutrient dense parts either. Fact: you can live well without regularly eating filler grains in your meals. Dark green vegetables like kale, spinach, collard greens, mustard greens, and other similar vegetables like cauliflower and broccoli, if eaten regularly, are going to give you all the complex carbs you need to give you a healthy dose of fiber and fuel from carbs.

Don't get me wrong. I love eating cereal and oatmeal, and I am not even saying they are unhealthy foods. Plenty of vegan athletes eat them in bulk and are successful at reaching their goals. I, thus far, have not been, and it sucks, because I especially love potatoes. Sweet potatoes are my favorite, but I learned the hard way about myself that when it comes to complex carbs, these starchy foods can be overkill if I want to get stronger without gaining fat.

The thing is, if you want to make your metabolism efficient at burning fat, it is going to need more practice at burning fat. It sounds so obvious it seems stupid, right? But relying on complex carbs for fuel all the time means you will either store fat until you can burn it (when you've burned through glycogen/carb storage), or you just end up having little to no need to consume fat on a regular basis. Of course, it can work the same way with fat—if you eat too many fat calories you will likely store more fat, and that is pretty easy to do because fat is the most calorically dense nutrient by 125% in comparison to carbs or protein. So the trick for me has been to eat the right amount of fat to fuel my daily activity and workouts. It took some experimentation, but I did figure it out.

Holistic dietitians and the Forks Over Knives doctors will tell you that you are best off avoiding fat and relying on complex carbs, but like I said earlier, being vegan is practically a failsafe for eating a ton of carbs and enough fiber. In fact, as a vegan, you're far more likely to eat too many carbs and too much fiber to gain muscle while also staying lean. Increasing fat intake is one way to slow the effect of all that fiber that is attached to complex carbs.

There is also an undeniable need for simple, sugary carbs too. These are the carbs that everyone is told ubiquitously to be "bad" carbs. These are the carbs that most often come from refined sugars or baked goods, meaning they are the ones that taste the fucking best, beyond all doubt. I pose the premise that perhaps there is no such thing as a bad carb, rather just bad times to eat certain types of carbs.

For example, after you've been working out for an hour or hour and a half, and your heart rate is up from kicking so much ass at lifting all that heavy-ass weight, and the glycogen storage in your muscles have been depleted by all the contractions and stress you've put your muscles through, there is no more opportune time to send your muscles a quick shot of glycogen-replenishing sugar. This could come in the form of a protein cookie, a smoothie with tropical fruit, dried fruit, yogurt, or even fruit juice. It could even be a motherfucking Pop Tart (strawberry flavor, no frosting, of course). The more simple the carb, the more quickly it will be digested and distributed back to the muscles which crave carbohydrates to be converted into glycogen. At this specific time in your day, complex carbs just won't do the trick (as well). They digest too slowly and take more energy from your already worn-out body to digest in that kind of situation. If you're ever going to eat simple carbs, do it right after you kick your own ass in a workout. The harder the workout, the more simple carbs you can enjoy. Earn those motherfuckers. They can make you fat when you're just sitting at work, especially if you eat more of them than you burn throughout the day, but immediate post-workout is a prime time to carb back up. I typically eat a Lenny and Larry's brand Protein Cookie after a heavy squat or deadlift day, right as I finish up, or sometimes I'll even eat a Lara Bar or banana. This kind of approach is detailed in the meal plan you will see later in the book.

I have eaten this way, by consuming sparse amounts of complex carbs via vegetables with my daytime meals and an ample dose of simple carbs immediately after my evening workout, for more than three years now, and not only has it helped me drop a weight class in competition, but I have also maintained that lower weight while gaining strength for the majority of the time, which all in all makes me a more competitive lifter. I also found this is an ideal way to enjoy eating junk food amid my otherwise very strict and healthy diet. Being able to eat these sugary foods on a near-daily basis helps me to not revert back to bad eating habits by creating cravings through deprivation.

Let's face it: we can all strive to be as healthy as possible and never eat junk food, but the reality is that the temptation sometimes becomes too great to avoid that cookie, or that brownie, or that ice cream, and by trying to be dietary saints we ripen the conditions for full-on junk food binges to befall us, which can ruin whatever results we had been working toward. To be able to work pliable dietary habits with both complex and simple carbohydrates into our repertoire is a more trustworthy foundation for long term success. Some people call this *flexible dieting*.

One last thing to consider about carbohydrates is that everyone's relationship to them varies by degree, and that is because of the finnicky hormone known as insulin, which is secreted by the pancreas to help transport sugar from food into cells for storage. If too much sugar is introduced into the bloodstream at once on a consistent basis insulin can become resistant, figuratively overwhelmed by excess blood sugar levels and cease to be effective in helping to convert and store sugar into cells for energy. This is how people develop Type-2 Diabetes.

But how much is too much? How much is unhealthy, and how much sugar will be eventually stored as fat? After all, our brains depend on glucose, as well as our muscles. So we need sugar, indisputably. And more importantly, when does insulin begin to cease to be effective at transporting sugar so it can be used as energy? That is the part of the equation that varies for everyone, and that everyone must likewise try to figure out on their own. To be sure, we've all met that guy or girl who eats doughnuts and sugary cereal every morning, then french fries for lunch, and some kind of burger or pizza for dinner, and somehow they look lean as hell. Yeah, fuck those lucky pricks. They seem to have perfectly sensitive insulin function despite all the simple and sugary carbs they overload themselves with. In a lot of ways that is just a lucky hereditary trait. Nevertheless, there are mindful ways and practices which can help the rest of us gauge and manage our insulin sensitivity.

The *glycemic index* refers to the rate at which carbohydrates are digested and effect blood sugar levels. Simple carbohydrates are generally digested the most rapidly, and therefore affect blood sugar levels more quickly, so they correspond to higher numbers on the glycemic index. Meanwhile, slower digesting complex carbs correspond to lower numbers on the index scale, because they affect blood sugar levels less rapidly. One example of one end of the spectrum of the glycemic index is refined sugar. On the complete other end, a leaf of dinosaur kale. In the middle towards the end of refined sugar there is dried fruit, like raisins. Also in the middle, but more towards the end with kale, is a sweet potato.

The idea behind the Vegan Meathead approach to carbs is to eat the complex ones sparingly during the day (in the form of vegetables) to store for energy, and then eat the simple ones in quick bursts when your metabolism is most apt to work hard and convert sugar in the blood to energy for the next day, that way excessive sugar does not linger in the bloodstream and increase insulin resistance. To be sure, there must always be *some* sugar in the bloodstream. To have too little blood sugar will cause you to faint, and this is why diabetics have to monitor their blood sugar levels. On the other hand, among the consequences of having too high a blood sugar level for too long are damaging small blood vessels, going blind, or losing your toes. Like with most things in life, balance is key.

Also important to note: simple carbs have little or no fiber, and thus tend to be absorbed or burned up very quickly. By this token, we can see that both types of carbohydrates are necessary at the appropriate times. For me, personally, I have found that eating slightly more fat calories than carb calories helps me keep the fat off by reducing the potentially overwhelming amount of fiber in a vegan diet and using fat as my primary fuel source. Some people, whom I envy, can handle more carbs than I can and still keep the fat off. It's a flexible balancing act no matter who you are, for sure, but the reward has been that I have been able to increase strength without gaining weight or fat composition for years now, and I don't even do cardio. I plan to keep this up, so I may never do cardio again. Amen.

PREFERRED SOURCES OF COMPLEX CARBS A.K.A DAYTIME CARBS

Berries (blueberries, strawberries, raspberries)

Dark Leafy Greens (kale, collard greens, mustard greens, spinach)

Green Vegetables (broccoli, cauliflower also qualifies)

PREFERRED SOURCES OF SIMPLE CARBS, GLUCOSE

*only to be consumed within one hour of end of workout

Lenny & Larry Protein Cookie

Lara Bar

Dried Fruit

Vegan Yogurt

Tropical Fruits (Banana, Pineapple, Mango)

DON'T BE A FAT-OPHOBE

SERIOUSLY, what is your problem? What is everyone's problem? Fat gets such a bad rap from everyone, but it does so many vital things to help you achieve Vegan Power, like: providing you with calories that aren't attached to fiber, providing you with calories that don't elevate blood sugar, and providing you with calories that won't require you to store extra glucose, which done in excess can make you fat.

This is all really important stuff. If you don't get good at burning fat, then yes, you will likely gain body fat unless you always eat at a significant caloric deficit, which will in turn restrict your ability to get stronger, and why even bother living if that's how you're going to go about it? The Way of The Vegan Meathead relies on more fat calories than carb calories, because believe it or not, it has proven for me to be the best way to keep fat off of my body. I found many other weightlifters and bodybuilders in my time who have said they have experienced the same thing in their relationship with fat.

Fat can be an amazing source of energy if you don't go overboard with fat calories, as each gram of it has more than double the calories of a gram of protein or carbohydrates. Of the three macronutrients, fat is gram for gram the most energy-potent by far. So make use of it!

After being taught to fear fat my whole life, I finally figured out that fat is much more simple to deal with than I ever anticipated—more simple than carbs by far. When it comes to fat in the Vegan Meathead meal plan, I keep it simple by limiting my main fat calories to a small handful of sources. There will always be more fat attached to other foods you eat, but those will be neglible sources compared to your preferred sources of fat.

PREFERRED SOURCES OF FAT:

Coconut Oil

Goddess Dressing (tahini sauce)

Vegan Mayonnaise (Vegenaise or Just Mayo brands)

Avocado

Nuts/Nut Butters (excluding pistachios, which are relatively low fat)

Note about Oils: While olive oil is technically a great source of fat, it does not hold up under the heat of a frying pan as well as coconut oil, so I opt for coconut oil every time I cook. Regarding coconut oil, I just use the refined blends, as the virgin blends are much more expensive and have that overwhelming coconut taste, which some people hate apparently.

PROTEIN SOURCES: TO ANSWER YOUR FUCKING ETERNAL QUESTION

AS I SAID EARLIER, *not all fake meats are created equally.* Just as this is also true for carbs, it is similarly true for protein powders. I have spent many years sorting through different plant-based protein products and fake meats. For lack of a better word, I do consider myself a sort of lay connoisseur in these matters, and after all this time I have developed a fierce loyalty to certain products and brands, simply because they have proven themselves to me by helping me in my goals. Much of this section will be a quick overlook of *the best* and *the decent* protein sources I am most familiar with: natural foods, powders, bars, and fake meats alike.

Please understand that the international market for plant-based protein products is growing so quickly that from the time I started writing this book until its publication, I can only estimate that there have been dozens if not hundreds of new plant-based formulas and brands launching game-changing products, many of which are likely outshining their predecessors in taste, texture, and overall quality. However, there is no way for me to include every new item I find in this book, so I just want to be clear that I am sticking to the items and brands that have actually helped me along my vegan strength path. There is no judgment, whether good, bad, or neutral, meant towards brands I was not able to include here. The way things are going, if I tried to include every protein powder, bar or pre-mixed shake option I can now find, I'd never finish writing this book. Luckily for you, this is the most exciting and convenient time to be vegan that we've seen yet, and it looks like it is only going to keep getting better.

The criteria for judging protein sources, as shown below, will be by *how many calories they require to give us one gram of protein*, of which the lower the number the better; what the *ratio of fiber is to one gram of protein*, of which the lower number is also better; and finally in the description below each title, I will mention what *percentage of protein per calorie* the food item holds (of which a higher number is better).

PROTEIN IN NATURAL FOODS

Some people will dislike what I am about to say, which is that natural food sources are not always the best sources of protein for vegans. Nevertheless, let's talk about some of the main ones, and why some are better than others.

TOFU

Calories per gram of protein: 9 (in extra firm tofu)
Ratio of fiber per gram of protein: 22%

Tofu really is the reigning king of natural protein sources, clocking in at 44% protein per calorie. This means that unless you have an actual soy allergy or intolerance, as a vegan, you better make friends with tofu. Tofu will do you right if you give it a chance.

Now, quite often I hear that people don't like tofu in dishes, because they either think it tastes like nothing, like a sponge, or they don't like the texture. Odds are these people haven't had tofu cooked well, and perhaps they don't even want to like it to begin with, but that is another issue entirely. Personally, I love tofu in many forms, fried especially, but no one cooks it better than restaurants with deep fryers, and who knows what kind of magic ingredients they are using in their fryers to make it so damn tasty. So as you will see in my meal plan in just a bit, I really don't cook and eat tofu in a chewable form often. Instead, I like to add it to my protein smoothies. Plain extra firm tofu adds a little thickness to a smoothie, while also adding a lot of protein with little interference in taste.

SEITAN

Calories per gram of protein: variably 5 to 7 (on average)
Ratio of fiber to gram of protein: 14 to 20% (on average)

If you're not familiar with seitan yet, get familiar. So long as you're not gluten-intolerant (you're more than likely not), seitan is going to play a key factor in your mission to achieve Vegan Power. Looking at the numbers above, you see I only listed a range for seitan's protein properties, and that is because every maker of seitan makes it slightly different. Being that seitan is typically just a beefy mix of wheat gluten with water and spices, density per batch and recipe can vary distinctly. You can even buy your own vital wheat gluten cheaply at the store, mix it with water and spices to your own preferences to make your own batches of seitan in minutes. It's very easy, but also kind of weird when you think about it, particularly when you are mixing that gummy wad of doughy wheat-based protein around on your counter until it becomes tough. I don't eat or make plain seitan often, but rest assured that it (errr, vital wheat gluten) is the prime ingredient of many Tofurky brand products that I practically live and thrive off of (which we'll get to shortly), and is why Tofurky items are often more dense than their other fake meat market competitor brands. One thing I will say is that if you eat a lot of Tofurky items you are basically eating a lot of seitan already, so making seitan dishes on your own will be less called for, just as eating a lot of soy protein bars, tofu, or fake meats with soy means supplementing with soy is also something I recommend avoiding. Ultimately, I do like to eat as many varied protein sources as possible, so if I already eat a lot of something I typically won't supplement with it, and vice versa.

TEMPEH

Calories per gram of protein: 10.5

Ratio of fiber to gram of protein: 54%

Tempeh is a traditional Indonesian soy food that is made from fermenting soybeans and binding them into a sort of cake form. It is also a great source of protein, iron, calcium, magnesium, and more, though people often complain about its slightly bitter or sour-ish taste. Again, that's their problem, and really they probably just need someone who knows what they are doing to prepare some for them to try. I love tempeh dearly, as it is a great well-rounded health food that boasts 38% protein per calorie, which is incredible, but I don't eat it as often tofu simply because of it's carb content and its flavor being incompatible with smoothies, as well as the fact that it is relatively high in fiber for a protein source, which decreases the bio-availability of amino acids in its proteins when digesting. Regardless, it's fun to incorporate tempeh into meals on occasion, namely with stir fry, sandwiches, or even breakfasts. Tofurky brand makes a delicious smoky maple tempeh.

BLACK BEANS

Calories per gram of protein: 16

Ratio of fiber to gram of protein: 74%

We are going to talk about black beans here as representatives for beans in general, primarily because they are among the top of the chain for protein-dense beans. A lot of people like to talk about beans being the essential source of protein for vegans and vegetarians, and while I agree that they are great for the average vegan or vegetarian, for a heavy weightlifter they are just not adequate to be the most dependable source of protein on a regular basis to feed muscles and build tissue, because as you can see, they are very high in fiber, meaning nearly as soon as you begin digesting them they are going to be on their way out of your system. And even at that, they are only about 24% protein per calorie, which is still high for the average person or food in general, but it's literally only about half as efficient at delivering amino acids to your muscles as tofu or seitan without factoring in the fiber and carbohydrate parts of the equation. In fact, black beans are typically three times richer in carbs than protein, so maybe consider a bean-heavy meal plan to carb up for long distance runs, but not if you want to be a Vegan Beast who lifts a lot of goddamn weight. Perhaps just enjoy them on occasion, as I do.

GREEN LENTILS

Calories per gram of protein: 10

Ratio of fiber to gram of protein: 100%

Green lentils, also known as split peas, are an interesting source of protein, as they boast a whopping 40% of protein per calorie, but they contain so much fiber (a gram for every gram of protein) that they are unarguably in the same boat as black beans in terms of bio-availability of proteins for absorption. It's all that goddamn fiber. I love lentils just like I love beans, but again, due to the high fiber content, I can't recommend them as a primary daily source of protein if you want to be competitive. Eat on occasion, and enjoy them when you do.

CHICKPEAS

Calories per gram of protein: 19

Ratio of fiber to gram of protein: 92%

Just like regular ol' beans, amateur vegans who don't lift talk about chickpeas (a.k.a garbanzo beans) like they are one of the greatest sources of protein around. Again, they taste great and are responsible for two of the best tasting offshoots of all time: falafel and hummus. And who doesn't like a hot plate of chana masala (Indian curried chickpeas)? You know I do. Love that shit. However, chickpeas fall into the lowest slot of protein category among their bean cousins, lentils and black beans, by only putting up 21% protein per calorie. Again, in the big picture of other foods in the world, that is still a lot of protein per calorie. Nevertheless, as badass and tasty as chickpeas are, they are not optimal sources of protein on a regular basis if you want to embark on The Way of The Vegan Meathead.

PROTEIN POWDERS

Unless you are one of the few random and gifted freaks of nature who possess the unusual trait of being able to self-synthesize enough protein in your body to satisfy the anabolic demands made by your workouts, or magically make use of the majority of protein you ingest from natural foods in spite of the fiber attached to them, it's a matter of necessity that you invest in some good vegan protein powder. Consider yourself unlucky, because you better believe that shit ain't cheap, but it is what it is, and if you want to make those gains you've been dreaming about that are going to save all the precious little piggies from gestation crates, you're going to need that protein to keep your metabolism busy without adding too many calories or grams of fiber.

So let us investigate which widely available protein powders in North America are the most efficient in terms of calories to protein, as well as bang for your buck, and most importantly, how good or terrible they taste. For the record, I am only reviewing proteins that I have actually used and that taste good enough to mix with water only. I don't mix protein powder with any kinds of milks, as that only adds useless calories, and if a protein blend doesn't taste good enough to chug when mixed with water only, I just don't bother. In my view, most proteins not featured on this list don't make the taste cut, though there are more any more brands and formulas popping up on the market every day now which I cannot humanly keep up with, so the exclusion of any specific brand or blend here does not mean I have any opinion about it, either way.

Also note, as I stated earlier, that I don't supplement with soy protein, because I eat a shit-ton of it, and consuming varied sources of protein is the responsible thing to do if you want to achieve Vegan Power, so there are no soy-based protein powders in the list of reviews.

NITROFUSION

Main protein sources: pea, artichoke, amaranth, quinoa
Calories per gram of protein: 5.7
Ratio of fiber to gram of protein: n/a
Average price: $59 for 5 pound tub
Cost per gram of protein: $.037
Taste: 8.5/10

NitroFusion is a protein line formulated by the PlantFusion company in New Jersey. It is almost the exact same product as PlantFusion, only with different packaging, and they seem to have substituted flax protein for artichoke protein (which will make no perceptible difference to your tastebuds), and more strangely, for some reason they don't seem to sell NitroFusion in stores, so it is only available to order online. One time at the Texas State Veggie Fair in Dallas I asked the sales rep at the PlantFusion table if I could buy any NitroFusion off of them, and she acted annoyed, retorting "You know it's practically the same thing as PlantFusion, right?" Yes, lady, I know, but NitroFusion is an overall better deal, and I go through a ton of this shit, so hook it up next time instead of being a brat. The best deal I have ever found online is Lucky Vitamin's $59 for a five pound tub with free shipping on top. Honestly, it's such an amazing deal that I only ever buy anything else if the shipment is taking longer than expected. NitroFusion is my shit. My favorite tasting protein powder, and thanks to Lucky Vitamin, the most cost efficient deal, too.

PLANTFUSION

    Main protein sources: pea, amaranth, quinoa, flax
    Calories per gram of protein: 5.7
    Ratio of fiber to gram of protein: n/a
    Average price: $32 for 2 pound tub
    Cost per gram of protein: $.051
    Taste: 8.5/10

As I stated above, PlantFusion and NitroFusion are practically the same thing. I really only buy PlantFusion when my big shipment of NitroFusion is out of stock from my online carrier and my shipment is delayed. In that case, I'll usually buy a one pound tub of PlantFusion at The Vitamin Shoppe or Whole Foods to hold me over for a week. Some people complain about the taste, citing that the sweetener tastes somewhat artificial, though it is just simple fructose. They used to use Stevia, I believe, as many powders also do, but it seems their formula keeps improving taste-wise if you ask me. PlantFusion is definitely one of the best deals if you are buying protein in a store.

SUNWARRIOR CLASSIC

Main protein sources: raw brown rice
Calories per gram of protein: 5.3
Ratio of fiber to gram of protein: 13%
Average price: $42 for 2.2 pound tub
Cost per gram of protein: $.060
Taste: 7/10

Sunwarrior brand provides some solid options. When I first started implementing protein powder into my diet about six years ago, I think Sunwarrior was one of the first brands I really latched on to. This particular line of Sunwarrior is only 15g of protein per scoop though, so you really need to put in 1.5 scoops per shake, and you go through the tub a lot faster that way. Also, because it is solely brown rice protein it is pretty damn chalky, but otherwise a solid option that has been championed by vegan lifters and bodybuilders for a long time.

SUNWARRIOR WARRIOR BLEND

Main protein sources: pea, hemp, goji berry
Calories per gram of protein: 5.5
Ratio of fiber to gram of protein: 5%
Average price: $45 for 2.2 pound tub
Cost per gram of protein: $.0625
Taste: 7/10

I'm a little torn on this item from Sunwarrior, as it isn't too much different overall from the Sunwarrior Classic, though the texture is less chalky, which is a good thing. You're basically spending about the same money for a blend that just tastes slightly different and comes from more varied protein sources. You'd just have to try them both to fairly know for yourself. I can honestly go either way if I am in a store where these two blends are my best options to choose from.

PLANT HEAD

Main protein sources: pea, brown rice, hemp, cranberry

Calories per gram of protein: 6

Ratio of fiber to gram of protein: 13%

Average price: $23 for 1.7 pound tub

Cost per gram of protein: $.051

Taste: 6.5/10

I've seen Plant Head coming up in a lot more shops over the past three or four years, and it is cool to have another quality all-raw protein blend to choose from. Admittedly, it does taste a bit like Sunwarrior Warrior Blend. The flavor is not too chalky, though it is kind of clumpy like dirt. The main problem with the product is that you really need to use 1.5 scoops to get 20 or more grams of protein per shake, and that makes the shake really thick, a texture that might be kind of gross for some people. I'm not too keen on that either, but when I need a dose of protein, I just say "fuck it" and get to chugging.

VEGA SPORT RECOVERY BLEND

Main protein sources: pea, pumpkin seed, sunflower seed, alfalfa
Calories per gram of protein: 5
Ratio of fiber to gram of protein: 6.7%
Average price: $45 for 1.81 pound tub
Cost per gram of protein: $.079
Taste: 7.5/10

Vega is a high quality company that has come a long way. I mean, Vega is just about in every major grocery store now, and it is even available at Target and Walmart. That's some keen business sense coming from some vegan Canadians. The thing that baffles me is that Vega, while a leader in its market, is not the best tasting, nor the most potent protein among its competitors, yet it is consistently the most expensive. Considering the amount of protein I go through consuming three shakes a day on normal days, whether I am in or out of the gym, price is a really big factor for me. So while I think Vega products have come a long way in taste, availability, and even in packaging, Vega is often a last resort for me. This Sport Recovery blend is marketed as having 30g of protein per serving, but that is only if you opt for the big serving, and that makes the shake a lot thicker and chalkier. It's not bad by any means, but I don't think the flavor is as good as PlantFusion or NitroFusion, and I really only buy this in individual packets at Whole Foods for $2 each or so when I just need to get through another day or two for my next batch of NitroFusion to come in.

VEGA CLEAN PROTEIN

Main protein sources: pea, hemp, pumpkin seed, alfalfa
Calories per gram of protein: 5.2
Ratio of fiber to gram of protein: 8%
Average price: $35 for 1.2 pound tub
Cost per gram of protein: $.093
Taste: 7.5/10

I feel very much the same way about this product as the one above, though I have never seen it in a large tub, so it is much more expensive compared to the other options I am reviewing here. If you're ever in a situation where you need protein, but this is your option, it'll do for sure, but it is going to cost you.

VEGA PROTEIN & GREENS

Main protein sources: pea, sacha inchi, hemp, brown rice
Calories per gram of protein: 6
Ratio of fiber to gram of protein: 10%
Average price: $40 for 1.79 pound tub
Cost per gram of protein: $.08
Taste: 8.5/10

Other than the Vega All One line, which is a meal replacement powder, I think the Protein & Greens line of Vega is the best tasting Vega stuff, easily. Again, it's just not the best deal per gram around, though it does have a great nutrient profile, and is easy to find in mainstream stores in case you're ever in a little protein emergency somewhere and need something of quality to hold you over.

MRM VEGGIE ELITE

    Main protein sources: pea, brown rice
    Calories per gram of protein: 5.4
    Ratio of fiber to gram of protein: 12.5%
    Average price: $32 for 2.4 pound tub
    Cost per gram of protein: $.044
    Taste: 7/10

This one is a catch-twenty two, as it is a really good deal, comparably, and it tastes pretty good, though it is made of rice and pea protein so it is notably chalky, but for some reason the mocha flavor of this brand gives me headaches. I genuinely like it and have bought it several times, but unlike other protein powders out there, it has given me mild headaches, and so I feel pretty weird about it. Maybe it's just me, but beware nonetheless.

ELEVATE PERFORMANCE PROTEIN

Main protein sources: pea, hemp, sacha inchi
Calories per gram of protein: 5.47
Ratio of fiber to gram of protein: 9.5%
Average price: $46 for 2-pound tub
Cost per gram of protein: $.073
Taste: 8/10

Elevate is a brand so new to the plant-based protein scene that it almost didn't make it in this book, but I tried it very recently and liked it so much I decided I'd have to include even though it is not widely available yet. And yeh, Disclaimer: I may be biased about it, as Elevate is owned and operated by my fellow PlantBuilt teammates, Paul and Jill Salomone. Despite knowing them personally and having great respect for them as vegan competitors and entrepreneurs, I can honestly and wholeheartedly tell you that the Elevate vanilla protein powder tastes great, and also boasts a competitive nutrient profile. I think in time this will be destined to become a popular brand for people seeking plant-based protein, as the blend has a nice smooth texture, a unique blend of protein sources, and an overall nutrient profile as good as any of my favorite proteins that I previously covered.

CLEAN MACHINE CLEAN GREEN PROTEIN WITH LENTEIN

Main protein sources: lentein, pea
Calories per gram of protein: 7.5
Ratio of fiber to gram of protein: 35%
Average price: $59.99 for 1.63-pound tub
Cost per gram of protein: $.15
Taste: 8/10

Clean Machine is a company doing new and interesting things. For example, their Clean Green Protein with Lentein ought to have you scrunching your forehead, asking "What the hell is Lentein?" According to their website, it is a lentil that grows in water. Well I'll be...

Clean Machine is a pack leader when it comes to offering high quality, nutrient dense, and high potency products. The only catch is that, yes, you are going to pay a pretty penny for them. Clean Machine's commitment to loading their protein powder full off other key nutrients like enzymes to increase absorption, super omegas, and green superfoods is commendable, but for someone who consumes as much protein as a strength athlete, it may prove financially difficult to consume a steady stream of this lentein-based mix (better work on getting a sponsorship!). It also has a high fiber to protein ratio, which makes me a little hesitant to invest so much into a powder like this on a regular basis, but the Vanilla Chai flavor smooth and tasty, though admittedly earthy (got that superfood aftertaste if you know what I mean), and it will make you poop green.

Ultimately, you will feel healthy as fuck on this stuff, and if you can afford it, Clean Machine is a unique and innovative brand that is bound to be bringing us game changing products to help us in our quest for vegan world domination. For discount codes, follow their social media or the many world class vegan atheletes they sponsor.

There you have it regarding some of the best vegan protein powders currently on the North American market. Note that I did not review Vega All One, Phood, or other meal replacement shakes because they are meal replacement shakes, not basic protein powders. I like to supplement protein, not replace meals. For strength I eat real meals. Bodybuilders often do meal replacement shakes to limit calories and maintain protein intake as they try to cut fat leading up to a competition. All I have to say about that is DIARRHEA. Stick to eating real food every day, supplement protein to meet your protein needs, and you'll be better off.

MEAT ANALOGS, A.K.A. FAKE MEATS

As I am typing this, there are food scientists cooking up ways to mimic meat in laboratory vats. They are doing this to create "real" meat for people to enjoy while removing the animal suffering, resource dilemmas, and environmental consequences from the equation of meat production. It's a noble endeavor, as I don't have a whole lot of faith in our species to collectively choose veganism outright, at least not on widespread cultural scales, so creating "real" meat in labs that does not have to come from the bodies of scared, trembling, tortured animals could go along way in bridging the gap between the kinds of behavior human beings *like* to engage in and the kinds of behavior we *ought* to engage in for ethical and rational reasons.

I have no doubt that the scientists cooking up these options for consumers will eventually succeed in creating a superior meat product, and they will make a fortune for helping save the world. Good for them. I applaud their ingenious efforts to circumvent rampant human apathy and stupidity. With that being said though, I think I will just stick with my tried and true meat analogs that I have been eating for years. For me personally, eating anything else that could more closely resemble real animal tissue in taste and texture than the products I am about to review for you would just be creepy. I am partial to the idea that I get to eat protein-dense food that is filling, tasty, and chewy, yet not quite like real murdered animal flesh. I know billions of people will feel differently, as they seem to prefer the taste, texture, and smell of dead carcasses, with ligaments, fatty gristle and all, but for now, as those "real" lab-made meats are not yet on the market, this section ought to help you discern your best options for "fake" meat, gram for gram, when you go to the store.

A little disclaimer: I am aware that in some more remote parts of North America, and for many readers outside of North America, the brands and items listed below are not readily available without the hassle and expense of mail or online ordering. I realize it is likely the same situation regarding the protein powders I reviewed as well. I know that in many parts of western Europe or Australia, for example, have their own burgeoning markets full of meat analog brands and protein powders. If, for anyone reading this, the mentioned products are not available, perhaps just use these reviews as a basis to compare the nutrient and macronutrient compositions of the brands available to you, or you can always refer back to the *Protein in Natural Foods* section to help mix and match to formulate a working meal plan for where you are, as tofu, seitan, tempeh, beans, lentils, and chickpeas are widely available and affordable virtually everywhere in the industrial world at this point. Now, onto fake meats that make the cut...

BEYOND MEAT

Currently, I think Beyond Meat is the leader of the pack of brands making awesome protein-dense fake meats that consistently taste excellent and have a ton of protein while not having too many carbs attached.

BEYOND CHICKEN GRILLED STRIPS

Calories per gram of protein: 6

Ratio of fiber to gram of protein: 10%

Percentage of protein per calorie: 66%

Looking at the numbers, you can see that Beyond Chicken Grilled Strips are a real winning product. Not only do they have one of the best protein profiles of any fake meat around, they are in my opinion among the tastiest too. As you'll see in my meal plan in a bit, I eat these for breakfast, usually dipped in a small amount of tasty fatty sauce, every damn day. Why anyone is still eating real murdered chickens, I have no idea. To add to their value, Beyond Meat routinely runs a $1 Off Coupon on their website every month. Print as many as you want and get $1 off each package of Beyond Meat you buy. Being that I eat this every day, you know I am printing off a shit ton of coupons.

BEYOND BEEF CRUMBLES

Calories per gram of protein: 7.5

Ratio of fiber to gram of protein: 15%

Percentage of protein per calorie: 52%

Not my absolute favorite Beyond Meat product, but a solid product nonetheless, especially good for making tacos, though when I usually eat these I really just heat them up with some green vegetables and use some Cholula hot sauce to spice things up and add flavor.

BEAST BURGER

Calories per gram of protein: 11

Ratio of fiber to gram of protein: 17%

Percentage of protein per calorie: 35%

The Beast Burger is an awesome burger patty in many ways, and though I do enjoy a Beast Burger now and then, there are a few reasons why I do not eat the Beast Burger, or burgers in general, on a regular basis. One reason is that a burger patty in itself is not a meal. You have to put condiments and buns on the thing to make it fully satisfying, and doing so adds a lot of useless calories that are bound to contain more sugar and fiber. Another reason is that the Beast Burger comes two patties to a box, and usually costs $5-$6, so that means they are not cheap, at least not for the amount of protein you get per dollar when compared to other options on this list. In defense of the Beast Burger though, it was crafted to contain a lot of iron and lot of Omega fatty acids, and that is a fair nutrient boost. Still, these are more of a treat on a cheat day than a regular in my rotation. As I am typing this, Beyond Meat is unveiling a new and potentially improved burger (the Beyond Burger) at select Whole Foods locations in the U.S., but I have not had it yet.

BEYOND BURGER

Calories per gram of protein: 14.5

Ratio of fiber to gram of protein: 15%

Percentage of protein per calorie: 28%

So I guess I get to be that guy. The guy who addresses the thing that everyone is raving about, and I tell you all: Guess what? It's not all *that* great. I am really sorry, folks. I hate being that guy, but I am just speaking from numbers here.

Okay, so saying the Beyond Burger is not all that great is harsh. But to be fair, I've been talking up Beyond Meat big time so far in this book (so much so that you may already think Beyond Meat is paying me to write this stuff, even if just in coupons… which unfortunately for me, they are not), so just know that what I am writing here is pure, honest criticism.

I sincerely don't mean to do any damage to one of the best fake meat companies in the game, nor any of their incredible products.

So let's get some things straight: the Beyond Burger is a great achievement in food science that is going to help animals because it is probably the closest thing to meat that people can buy in the grocery store at the moment that isn't actual dead animal flesh. The way Beyond Meat is marketing this product is brilliant, having it in the actual meat section and all. The beet coloring that they have emphasized in the recipe even makes it look like real beef patties, and while that grosses me out a little bit, I bet most shithead North Americans will be amped about that. Everything Beyond Meat has done to market this burger is a fucking power move, and I hope they make tens of billions of dollars off of it.

But here's the thing everyone who is serious about eating for strength needs to know: as far as nutritional profile goes, the Beast Burger is a superior burger to the Beyond Burger, even if only negligibly. The Beast Burger has less calories and more protein, straight up. You might like the way the Beyond Burger tastes more than the Beast Burger, and you may even like the softer texture of the Beyond Burger too, and those are all fair preferences, but that's just not what I care about ultimately. The Way of the Vegan Meathead always considers the bottom line, and the bottom line here is which burger gives you more protein per calorie, and there is no arguing with the fact that the Beyond Burger is not that burger.

Besides, if you're eating to become a lean Vegan Beast, burgers are not every day food, because they always require extra calories from condiments and buns to complete the package, so this whole conversation about the better burger is moot. You ought to be eating Beyond Chicken strips every day of the week for the most part, and reserve either burger for party time on the weekend.

TOFURKY

Tofurky is the other undisputed heavyweight of vegan meat brands, and truly I can't say enough good things about Tofurky, as they are a true pioneer in the market of fake meats—so much so that Tofurky is synonymous with what vegetarians eat on Thanksgiving, whether they are actually eating Tofurky or not. A true household name. While they gained popularity with their now infamous Holiday Roast, a gluten-laden ball of veggie protein stuffed with wild rice and made to appeal to former turkey-eaters, they have gracefully branched out to make everything from sausage to "chick'n" to pizza, hot pockets, quiche, and more. All the employees of Tofurky I have met have been truly warm and kind people, including the Tibbott brothers who started the Tofurky brand over thirty years ago from very humble origins with a vision to help animals by improving vegetarian food options.

TOFURKY ITALIAN SAUSAGE
Calories per gram of protein: 9
Ratio of fiber to gram of protein: 3%
Percentage of protein per calorie: 43%

Tofurky's Italian Sausage is one of the easiest vegan sausages to find just about anywhere, and it is one of the best deals around too. I usually buy a package of four links for $2.50 to $4 each, depending on the store, meaning each link that contains 30 grams of protein costs a dollar or sometimes much less. Considering that I eat two of these a day, most days per week, that's really good news for me. These, along with Beyond Chicken Grilled Strips, are my go-to protein sources for the first half of my day.

Tofurky does have other flavors of sausages like Kielbasa, Beer Brats, Chick'n and Apple, Cajun Andouille, Spinach and Pesto, and a couple other I believe, but none of them have quite as much protein (though to be fair, they still have a lot), and because they seem to be less popular and therefore less widely distributed, they are usually a little more money. Besides, I think the Italian flavor is the best.

TOFURKY DELI SLICES

Calories per gram of protein: 7.5

Ratio of fiber to gram of protein: 23%

Percentage of protein per calorie: 52%

Tofurky Deli Slices come in a variety of flavors, from Oven Roasted (my personal favorite), Hickory Smoked, Peppered, and Bologna. These deli slices, to me, are not best suited to be meals because generally they'd need to be part of a sandwich to make something truly filling. They are of course great for going on a road trip and making sandwiches for an occasion like that, but on a regular basis I mostly indulge in them for a late night, high protein snack. I may dip them slice by slice, breadless, into hummus or lightly into a vegan mayo. For only 100 calories they do give a good shot of protein to keep your metabolism busy before and during bedtime.

TOFURKY SLOW ROASTED CHICK'N
Calories per gram of protein: 8
Ratio of fiber to gram of protein: 7%
Percentage of protein per calorie: 49%

These are among the newest of Tofurky products, and I must say they are top notch. All the flavors are excellent, from Lightly Seasoned to Thai Basil to Sesame Garlic, Barbecue, or Tandoori. Tofurky Slow Roasted Chick'n has become a great way to mix up my usual routine of eating Italian Sausage twice a day most days a week. I usualy reserve this option for days where I am lifting heavier than usual, because these products are slightly more calorically-dense than the sausages. That's perfectly okay on days where I can use an extra energy boost though.

TOFURKY HOLIDAY ROAST
Calories per gram of protein: 7.5
Ratio of fiber to gram of protein: 15%
Percentage of protein per calorie: 53%

The cornerstone of Tofurky products. You used to see these things exclusively sold around Thanksgiving or Christmas, but now they seem to be so popular I am seeing them everywhere all the time. Gardein also makes a comparable stuffed holiday roast, and it is good, but Tofurky will always be my favorite. While I don't eat this routinely much of the year, I am always looking forward to the time of the year where I can eat it many days straight with my family and then for leftovers. Typically speaking, this roast also calls for gravy or cranberry sauce to be eaten with it, and those calories were not factored into the calculations I made here. More than anything, when eaten with the proper side dishes and condiments accompanying it, this is more of an occasional treat than a staple.

GARDEIN

I've got to hand it to Gardein for being one of the most innovative and prolific vegan meat companies out there, if not the most. They have so many varieties of vegan meats and flavors that I can't even keep up with them all, and more than likely, whichever store you shop at will only have a select few based on local popularity. It is certainly near impossible to get bored with the smorgasbord that is Gardein brand.

The only flip side regarding Gardein is that their meats are typically not quite as protein-dense as those of Beyond Meat or Tofurky, and their products rely heavily on sauces for flavor—meaning more sugar and carbs from the sauces. This doesn't mean it's never a good time to eat Gardein items, but it does mean I try to be more selective about when I eat them.

I definitely don't eat them every day like I usually do with Tofurky or Beyond Meat. Nevertheless, please don't take that as me saying you shouldn't enjoy Gardein's goodness semi-often. You should.

Here is just a sliver of the selection Gardein offers, most of which are my favorites, but be advised that they have many other comparable items to these that are similar in both taste and protein profile.

SWEET AND SOUR PORKLESS BITES

Calories per gram of protein: 10.5

Ratio of fiber to gram of protein: 15%

Percentage of protein per calorie: 38.5%

*calculated by using half packet of sauce

These are pretty much my favorite Gardein product, as it is one of the few with about equal carbs to protein, and it tastes fucking excellent. Again, the taste comes from the sauce, and to be honest, it's more sauce than anyone needs, so I regularly only use half a packet on the whole bag of bites. I usually only eat these for dinner on an occasional day off from the gym.

BEEFLESS TIPS

Calories per gram of protein: 9
Ratio of fiber to gram of protein: 16%
Percentage of protein per calorie: 45%

Another great option to eat in place of the Porkless Bites on the occasion of eating a basic meal on a day off from the gym. Great flavor, no extra sauce to mix either. Very filling.

SWEET AND TANGY BARBECUE WINGS

Calories per gram of protein: 9
Ratio of fiber to gram of protein: 14%
Percentage of protein per calorie: 43%
*calculated by using full packet of sauce

Well, if you're going to eat wings, you know it is necessary to not skimp on the sauce. These take longer to do correctly because they require oven use. When you do them in the microwave you are doing them a disservice.

TERIYAKI CHIK'N STRIPS

Calories per gram of protein: 10
Ratio of fiber to gram of protein: 14%
Percentage of protein per calorie: 40%
*calculated by using half packet of sauce

A solid option. No need to use all the sauce. As you can see, the protein profile doesn't come close to Beyond Meat's chicken strips, but you know, sometimes you just need to lighten up. Not too often, but sometimes.

CHIPOTLE LIME CRISPY FINGERS

Calories per gram of protein: 13
Ratio of fiber to gram of protein: 13%
Percentage of protein per calorie: 30%

These are so good they require no sauce, but since they are breaded you run into the carb/sugar trap. I love these, but eat them sparingly.

CHIK'N SLIDERS

    Calories per gram of protein: 18
    Ratio of fiber to gram of protein: 10%
    Percentage of protein per calorie: 22%
    *calculated without considering the amount of calories added to these numbers by using condiments.

Honestly, these are just a guilty pleasure. Put some Chao brand vegan cheese on them, and maybe some chipotle vegan mayo. Man, they're too fucking good, so I really have to guard myself against these. These are a total cheat-day-only kind of entree, especially with all the other condiments I like to add. They're just so tasty, so be careful.

MEATLESS MEATLOAF

    Calories per gram of protein: 12.5
    Ratio of fiber to gram of protein: 26%
    Percentage of protein per calorie: 31.5%
    *calculated by using full packet of sauce

You know... it's meatloaf, so it's not the greatest thing ou've ever eaten, but it's nice to mix it up and have it as an option, as these are great despite being "meatloaf." You definitely need to use all of the sauce packets on these otherwise they are just too dry.

FIELD ROAST GRAIN MEAT CO.

Field Roast has the unfavorable stigma of appearing to be a sort of underdog little brother to Tofurky's sausage and wheat meat empire, but I must say that Field Roast undeniably makes some products which altogether hold their own to make them one of the best vegan meat companies out there. One issue they face, at least in terms of me personally buying their products, is that since they seem to not be quite as popular as Tofurky, they are distributed less commonly and cost significantly more. For example, a pack of Tofurky sausages will on average cost between $3 and $4, while a pack of Field Roast sausages costs around $5.50. That discrepancy adds up if you are constantly eating vegan sausage. Despite the cost factor, when I do get Field Roast products, it is always worth it, as they truly have superlative products.

SMOKED APPLE SAGE SAUSAGE

Calories per gram of protein: 9.25

Ratio of fiber to gram of protein: 11.5%

Percentage of protein per calorie: 43%

As much as I love Tofurky Italian Sausage, this particular sausage right here is by far the best tasting one on the market, and I know many people who agree. This smoked apple sage sausage by Field Roast is a delight of a delight. Like I said, it's going to cost you a little more than Tofurky Italian Sausage, and it's doesn't have quite as much protein either, but every now and then it is nice to splurge and enjoy these bad boys, because they are as tasty as it gets.

Field Roast's other sausages, the Chipotle Mexican and the Italian flavors, are also good but have even less protein than this one. Also, if you don't like fennel seeds, steer clear of the Italian Field Roast sausage as it has quite a bit of them. That seems to be an acquired taste for a lot of people, and for me, between Field Roast Italian Sausage and Tofurky Italian Sausage, it's no contest. Tofurky wins that one by a long shot in both value and taste. If you're going to get Field Roast sausage, this Smoked Apple Sage flavor is the one to get.

APPLE MAPLE BREAKFAST SAUSAGE

Calories per gram of protein: 10

Ratio of fiber to gram of protein: 20%

Percentage of protein per calorie: 40%

These lil puppies are one of the best options to accompany a nice cheat day breakfast of pancakes. Imagine that: sausages that almost taste like dessert. So fucking good, and one package makes 50 grams of protein. Try to not eat the whole thing at once! Best to share.

LENTIL SAGE DELI SLICES

Calories per gram of protein: 7
Ratio of fiber to gram of protein: 14%
Percentage of protein per calorie: 56%

Field Roast has managed to make deli slices that beat Tofurky's deli slices by protein profile. Taste-wise they are similar to Tofurky but more nuanced and fancy, as sometimes there are noticeable pieces of lentils in the slices which adds a texture to them that some people will enjoy and others will not. The only drawback is that they are harder to find and cost more. Sometimes it is worth it though. Definitely put these in your rotation from time to time as a late night protein snack that requires no preparation.

CELEBRATION ROAST

Calories per gram of protein: 9
Ratio of fiber to gram of protein: 19%
Percentage of protein per calorie: 44%

You could say this is the closest thing to a competitor to Tofurky's holiday roast on Field Roast's roster, as it is a one-pound ball of protein stuffed with mushrooms, apples, and butternut squash. Being that these things aren't normally sold frozen like Tofurky roasts, they require less prep time and are easy to just slice up and fry with a little oil in a pan for an outstanding protein-filled dinner any time of the year. Absolutely delicious and guaranteed to keep your stomach busy digesting for hours because you won't know when to stop eating this thing. Major props to Field Roast for putting apples in everything to make their products so fucking tasty. Nice trick, fellas!

SWEET EARTH NATURAL FOODS

Sweet Earth is not an all-vegan company, but they do churn out some great vegan products that are becoming widely available nonetheless. I have enjoyed their curry seitan and other seitan products before. Their beefy seitan crumbles are good but not as protein-dense as Beyond Meat Beef Crumbles and I can't get regular coupons for them, so I don't ever opt for them. I know their veggie burger patties seem to be catching on with a lot of people, as are a lot of the frozen meals, which may or may not be vegan. What I enjoy Sweet Earth best for though is their Benevolent Bacon.

BENEVOLENT BACON

Calories per gram of protein: 9

Ratio of fiber to gram of protein: 10%

Percentage of protein per calorie: 44%

The best vegan bacon on the market, hands down. Fry it up with some coconut oil and you are GOOD. Also an obvious partner for that cheat day breakfast of pancakes if you ain't in a mood for sausage.

PROTEIN BARS

By now you may be thinking, "But Daniel, we've got the tofu and the Tofurky, and the Beyond Meat and the Gardein, and the protein powder. Now you're saying we have to get protein bars, too?"

Uhhh yes. Of course I am telling you exactly that. This book is called The Way of The Vegan Meathead. It's not *The Way of The Salad-Eating, Meditating Hippie Vegan.* I expect you to eat to accommodate dominant lifting habits. I want you to become stronger than me, stronger than any other vegan before, and most definitely stronger than all those omnivore dickheads out there. To do that you're going to need significant quantities of protein in nearly everything you eat, all the damn time, including your pre- and post-workout snacks. That is where protein bars come into the equation, so let's get to know your best options.

CLIF BUILDER'S BAR

Calories per gram of protein: 14

Ratio of fiber to gram of protein: 20%

Percentage of protein per calorie: 28.5%

There was a time when these things were hard to find. It becomes increasingly harder to recall that time with each new day, as Builder's Bars become more popular and more available everywhere you go, from the most remote gas station along the most desolate highways in parts of America that feel eerily post-apocalyptic, to the most decadent supermarkets in the yuppiest gentrified neighborhoods imaginable. You bet your ass they've got Builder Bars, and people are so busy gobbling them down they don't even realize they are technically vegan.

In fact, most of the Clif Bar empire is vegan, though they don't market it as such, and there are unfortunately some exceptions, like Builder's MAX bars, and Luna Protein bars, which have added whey. For all the frivolous crying that so much of the consumer public does about soy being toxic or causing men to grow women's breasts (which is all ridiculous, to be sure), people sure seem to love these Clif brand bars that are made almost entirely out of soy protein isolates.

To be perfectly candid with you, I think the Chocolate Peanut Butter flavor of Builder's Bar is one of the finest delicacies ever crafted. If I ever find myself on Death Row for this or that, and I am afforded the rite of a last meal, I am just going to ask for a box of Builder's Bars. When I finish a dozen of them, I ought to be feeling so good I'll be ready to go in peace. They are drug-like in how good they taste. Thank Odin they are technically vegan.

Now, just to be clear, I don't eat more than one Builder's Bar a day, and even then I only eat them on days I lift. They actually have a lot of carbs and a lot of calories. One bar has about as many calories as one of my small lunch meals, so what I like to do is utilize the carbs from this bar by eating about an hour or hour and a half before I hit the gym. This is a low glycemic treat, believe it or not, so it is really more fitting to describe these bad boys as energy bars than prime sources of protein.

NUGO SLIM BAR

Calories per gram of protein: 10.5
Ratio of fiber to gram of protein: 41%
Percentage of protein per calorie: 38%

I can't lie. I love chocolate, and the dark chocolate crunchy peanut butter bar by NuGo Slim is the next best thing to a Builder's Bar on my days off when I need to be eating less calories. At 17 grams of protein per bar, these babies make just right for a tasty little snack on the way home from work. They have a lot of goddamn fiber though, so more than anything they are a treat for those of us with a sweet-tooth. Get some protein with your sweet treats, alright? The soy protein isolate that makes up the bulk of the body of this bar is pretty gritty, but that dark chocolate coating hits the spot just right.

BASE PROTEIN BAR (BY PRO BAR)

Calories per gram of protein: 14.5
Ratio of fiber to gram of protein: 20%
Percentage of protein per calorie: 27.5%

Pro Bar, as a company, rose to popularity by selling it's meal replacement bars. They have more recently tried to get into the protein bar game, facing off most directly with Clif Builder's Bar. The Base Protein Bar by Pro Bar is honestly just a Builder's Bar that doesn't taste quite as good, has a grittier protein mix noticeable in the body of the bar, a slightly inferior protein profile, but somehow costs almost twice as much on average. It's nice to have another protein bar on the market with different flavors than the ones Builder's Bar offers, but overall this is not the best deal or best tasting bar. I really only buy them when they are on clearance.

ELEVATE PROTEIN BAR

Calories per gram of protein: 12.9

Ratio of fiber to gram of protein: 52%

Percentage of protein per calorie: 29.6%

The only flavor of protein bar Elevate is currently selling is Chocolate Chip Cookie Dough, and it very comparable in taste and texture to a MetRX bar (not vegan), if you recall those. The Elevate bar has slightly less calories than the Clif Builder bar, and the same amount of protein, but it is significantly higher in fiber, which is problematic for a protein bar. It has even more fiber than the NuGo Slim bar, too. The primary protein source in this bar, though, is pea protein isolate, unlike any of the other bars on this list, which are all soy protein based. It's nice to see a company sourcing protein isolate other than soy for its base, for variety if no other reason, as some people will want to opt for a bar without soy in it. These are also currently much more expensive than any of their protein bar competitors, but I expect to see that price go down as Elevate becomes more popular as a brand.

LENNY & LARRY'S COMPLETE PROTEIN COOKIE

Calories per gram of protein: 26
Ratio of fiber to gram of protein: 37.5%
Percentage of protein per calorie: 15%

All things considered, the Complete Protein Cookie by Lenny & Larry is not exactly a protein *bar*, per-se. Indeed, as the title reads, it is a cookie. It is advertised primarily as a source of protein, but it's really just a carb overload that's sufficient as a post-workout treat because it has some protein too. That, and they are damn good, but at any other time of the day these things will make you fat unless you're one of the lucky kinds of pricks with an inhuman junk-burning metabolism that I mentioned earlier. But you know how we talked about insulin and the proper time to eat simple carbs? This is where Lenny & Larry come in big for a strength athlete.

At 400 calories per cookie, the only time you can justify eating a whole one of these things is when you've just finished a historically brutal session. I mainly save these for my deadlift or squat days when I am doing reps at or over 85% of my max. Get the sugar into your blood quick to get that glycogen back in your muscles after you have destroyed them.

You only get 16 grams of protein out of the whole damn cookie, which is a snack at any other time of the day, but considering all the carbs and sugar attached, it'd otherwise be pure sacrilege to your fitness lifestyle if not for the timing of its consumption. *Then and only then*, right after you have annihilated yourself, eating one of these can be justified.

Be careful, too, because Lenny & Larry do not run an entirely vegan company (yet, anyway), and all of the other products they sell are not vegan. For now, only the cookies are legit.

NOT-ENOUGH-PROTEIN BARS

There are a lot of so-called "protein bars" out there that know-nothings regard as protein bars, so let's just take a quick moment to review some bars that are merely snack bars or quick energy bars, and in reality are nowhere close to being adequate protein bars (and are therefore useless in most circumstances).

For the consistency of our protein bar litmus test, let's set the standard for all relevant protein bars at a minimum of 15 grams per bar. I'd say that's a very lenient standard, but henceforth, if a bar does not meet that 15 gram requirement, it it will officially be called a *Not-Enough-Protein Bar.*

CLIF BAR

Calories per gram of protein: 25

Ratio of fiber to gram of protein: 70%

Percentage of protein per calorie: 16%

Example One: perhaps the most popular Not-Enough-Protein Bar of all time, the Clif Bar.

At a measly 9-10 grams per bar (depending on the flavor), the Clif Bar costs you 250 calories, a ton of sugar, but not much yield on long-burning muscle-feeding amino acids. For 30 more calories you can get double the protein and a dose of slow-burning low glycemic energy in a Builder's Bar. If you're going to go run 15 miles, consider eating a Clif Bar. If you're going to lift heavy-ass weight and back down to no one, the Clif Bar just became irrelevant to you.

LUNA BAR

Calories per gram of protein: 25

Ratio of fiber to gram of protein: 50%

Percentage of protein per calorie: 16%

Who would have thought that a "protein bar" marketed at women would have the same protein profile and even less fiber (which, remember, is a good thing if you want more time to absorb amino acids)? I didn't even realize that until I made these computations for this book. From now on if I am in a life or death starvation situation in the middle of fucking nowhere, and my only options in the gas station are Clif Bars or Luna Bars, you can bet I will be choosing the Luna Bars.

Also, ladies primarily, beware of Luna Protein bars, a newer line by Luna that has an extra two or so grams of protein. Those are not vegan as they have whey as the added protein. Stupid.

LARA BAR

Calories per gram of protein: 38
Ratio of fiber to gram of protein: 50%
Percentage of protein per calorie: 10.5%

I am fairly sure no one in their right mind, except maybe my wonderful mother, has ever thought a Lara Bar was a protein bar, but just to be clear since they are always next to protein bars in stores, Lara Bars are most definitely Not-Enough-Protein Bars. In fact they are almost entirely just dehydrated fruit, which is essentially CANDY, which is pure sugar. There is no time ever that one following The Way of The Vegan Meathead should ever eat a Lara Bar, except for a little glucose boost during an exceptionally long workout, or right after a workout, perhaps when a Complete Cookie is not available, or when a workout was not punishing enough to warrant eating the amount of carb-based calories in a Complete Cookie. Other than that, stay clear of these things. This is runner's food.

NUGO DARK BAR

Calories per gram of protein: 20
Ratio of fiber to gram of protein: 10%
Percentage of protein per calorie: 20%

So...these things taste good. They aren't as lousy as Clif or Luna Bars, but all in all, they are still Not-Enough-Protein Bars, and there is no talking their way out of it. 10 grams of protein is virtually nothing, especially if it costs 200 calories. Nuff said.

PRIMAL STRIP

Calories per gram of protein: 8
Ratio of fiber to gram of protein: 10%
Percentage of protein per calorie: 49%

I was really unsure where to put Primal Strips. Are they more like protein bars, or not-enough-protein bars? They don't have 15 grams of protein, but they are also usually 100 calories or less (each flavor can vary quite a bit) and offer nearly 50% protein per calorie, as they are basically ultra-saucy strips of seitan or soy isolate. I think the best I can do for Primal Strips is put them at the end of the bars section here, and suggest them as an occasional snack. I do love the flavors of these things and they are a good little dose of protein for something that is relatively low calorie, but at the same time they just aren't significant enough in their overall sustenance to count as anything else. You could eat two of them for a significant boost of protein and still be under 200 calories, but price-wise this does not make as much sense as most other actual protein bars I discussed.

Other vegan bars that qualify as Not-Enough-Protein bars: *GoMacro* bar (11g protein, 240 cal), and *Chia Bar* (4g protein, 100 cal). I am sure there are others, but really, who fucking cares? Sorry folks, they just have too many calories and too little protein. If you want lean vegan gains, I cannot recommend these. Just because something is vegan and has some protein doesn't mean it works for this program.

Side Note about Meal Replacement Bars: I decided to not review meal replacement bars, like *Pro Bar MEAL* bars, just like I decided to not review meal replacement powders, because they don't fit into our overall goal of eating an efficient balance of protein to overall calories. Meal replacement bars have way too many calories for the protein they offer. A 320-400 calorie "meal" needs to offer you at least 30g protein to be adequate. Don't take it the wrong way, meal-replacers, we're just not compatible, and it isn't your fault.

SNACKS

While we are on the subject of piddly-ass foods that aren't going to do anything for you but make you get pudgy or float around like a fairy, maybe both (ever heard of skinny-fat?), let's talk about snacks.

In the Vegan Meathead meal plan that I am sure you already skimmed forward to, you will see that there really isn't much room for snacks. Snacks are not factored in to the schedule because you are normally eating every two to two and a half hours. Though you will mostly be eating small meals that are around 300 calories, and on occasion a little more, you really shouldn't be getting so hungry that you need a little something in between all those meals, smoothies, and shakes.

However, knowing that you are a human being, and it is merely in your DNA to disobey, smite, and disappoint the gods, let's go over some snacks that won't get you in to too much trouble.

#1 Best Snack: Water

You read that right. Just drink more water. Exciting, huh? You bet I just tricked you, except I am helping you, I swear. Water staves off hunger as good as anything else, it's good for those protein-filtering kidneys, and it costs you no calories. Drink water all goddamn day or keep your weak lifestyle forever. Your choice. You were hoping for soda? Fuck you.

#2 Best Snack: Nuts

Now, like other things we've talked about, not all nuts are created equal, but the nuts that will suffice on a fairly equal level to each other are almonds, walnuts, cashews, and peanuts. All pathetically juvenile jokes aside, the thing that is tricky about nuts is that they are small and easy to eat a lot of, especially if you are starving, and since they have so much fat the calories can add up fast without even realizing it. So the thing I like to do is get those Emerald brand 100-calorie packs of whichever kind of nuts they have at the store (Trader Joe's also offers their own brand of these). Opt for unsalted and as natural and raw as you can, because you want as many of those 100 calories to come from fat or protein as possible.

#3 Best Snack: Cup of Coffee

You've got to watch out about drinking too much coffee (or caffeine, to be specific), as more than a few 8-ounce cups of caffeinated coffee a day can potentially lead toward chronic dehydration, or raise blood pressure—neither of which will be good for you as lifter, or as a human animal. However, if you only have a couple cups a day you ought to be fine. I have one cup in the morning usually, and then I like to have another one an hour or thirty minutes prior to working out to help get myself psyched to lift. Plus, that warm feeling in the belly that coffee gives you will help you feel less hungry for a little bit while costing you no calories (or just negligible calories if you are using some plant-based creamer or milk—don't overdo it with the creamer or milk though!). I suppose tea could work in place of coffee too, but for whatever reason I usually feel more full from coffee. Maybe that's just me...

As far as snacks go, that's all you get! Get used to sticking to the meal plan since I already worked in protein bars as snacks. There really should be little to no room for you to be hungry between shakes and meals.

One other important thing to consider is that it is okay to feel hungry sometimes. Unless you have an eating disorder of some kind, it is even *necessary*. If you eat small meals often (as according to the meal plan) with the goal of keeping fat off or burning fat, hunger is bound to happen. So get used to those pangs now and then. You just don't want to feel hungry for a prolonged amount of time on a regular basis, as that is when your metabolism will start burning up muscle mass. We're not starving ourselves here, just rationing wisely. There is a big difference, being that it is very possible and realistic to make continual gains while eating at a slight caloric deficit.

SUPPLEMENTS

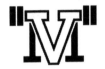

RIGHT OFF THE BAT I must say: don't be one of those whiny assholes who swears up and down that "all you'll ever need to be strong and healthy is in plant-based whole foods." I'm serious. You're not helping anyone when you say that shit. It's just fucking annoying, and for the most part it's only true if the most extensive exercise you're going to do is jogging at the park, or riding your bike on a flat street, or doing jumping jacks or some other form of 'warm-up' exercises. I will concede to you that if your goal is to be 'slim' and reduce your chances of developing chronic disease, then yes, sticking to the plant-based whole foods path is a perfectly acceptable route to take. But like I have been saying, if you want to be a Vegan Beast, you've got to literally annihilate your body multiple times a week for years, and that process of destroying and reconstructing your muscles and increasing bone density takes more than adequate calories, minerals, amino acids, and vitamins to heal and be better than before. The bottom line: just accept that you will need some supplements to facilitate the healing, growth and maintenance to achieve ambitious goals. Juicing and miso really only go so far.

The good news is that you really don't need an overflowing bounty of supplements to ensure you put your body on the right path, and even better, most of the ones I will recommend to you are relatively inexpensive. The biggest investment required out of all of them is your quality protein powder, which is first and foremost. Since we have already covered some of the best vegan protein powder options on the market right now, this section is going to focus on minor supplements that are typically optional for you (depending on what your goals are), though there are select ones that I judge to be non-optional.

NON-OPTIONAL SUPPLEMENTS

Vitamin B12

If there's one vitamin you need to be sure to take as a vegan, it is B12. Do not fuck this one up. If there is one piece of pivotal information I'd prefer you to remember from this entire dazzling work of bro-art you are reading, it's that you better be taking your B12. Why? Because no matter who you are, whether you are an aggressive athletic vegan, a yoga mom, or a pitiful omnivore, B12 is an notoriously difficult vitamin to absorb.

If you look at the nutrition facts of any B12 product you will see that each serving is usually thousands or tens of thousands of percent higher than the recommended daily value.

That's because B12 is actually a bacteria that is very resistant to being absorbed, and aside from the revolting secretions and flesh of murdered animals, there are no foods that naturally provide a significant amount of B12. You can take 16,000% of your RDV of B12 a day, and it would still be possible to not absorb 100% of your estimated needs. So take B12 everyday, perhaps twice if you are going to have a heavy deadlift or squat day, because one of the primary functions of B12 is to support basic central nervous system (CNS) health, and if you are deficient in B12 long enough you can cause permanent damage to nerve cells. That would be a fucking disaster, and think of how many precious animals you *won't* be saving by not inspiring people to go vegan. You need to recruit motor function and have all your neurons firing smoothly to rip that bar off the floor for a new PR, or come up hard out of the hole on a death-defying squat.

A little anecdote for ya: For the first 5 or so years as a vegan I did not ever take B12. I actually took no supplements. I was really skinny back then, and at best my inconsistent exercise habits included running, pull-ups and push-ups. That was about it. I never pushed my body to any sort of limits, especially not my central nervous system. Sometime around late 2010, 5 years into my vegan path, I decided to get serious about achieving Vegan Power, and I began learning to squat and deadlift properly, as well as learn ways to ambitiously improve my bench press. Within about six months I would notice mental fatigue during or after workouts. Once I got my deadlift up to about double my bodyweight I would often see stars or be faint for a moment after pulling. I remember the night I first pulled 300 pounds at a bodyweight of about 150. It was a big achievement for me back then, hitting that double-bodyweight mark, but

I swear I nearly passed out once I set that weight back down. I realized that week that I had reached a point of danger in my lifting ambitions, so I needed to look into ways of maintaining myself better. I soon began taking B12 regularly. The fortunate thing is that from point on, light-headedness from lifting ceased to happen. Sure, maybe there are many explanations for that. Maybe I simply conditioned my CNS to adapt by lifting heavier and heavier over time, but considering that I had never taken B12 before in my life, it's reasonable to think that building up my B12 storage was at least helpful to my conditioning.

I have a friend who has never taken B12. He's been vegan more than 20 years at this point, who overall eats decently, but is not a heavy lifter, and he is notoriously known by all our other friends for being the guy who is always falling asleep, like Abe Simpson, bordering on narcolepsy. He refuses to take B12 simply because I told him he should. Meanwhile he's doing terrible PR for veganism and the animals when he falls asleep in front of everyone all the time. Maybe he gets by in his overall health with the B12 in fortified almond or soymilk, or cooking with nutritional yeast. It's hard to be sure how, but we're not here to just get by, so don't be like him, alright? We're going to attract new people to the vegan team by displaying our power and vitality, and that means taking your B12.

Vitamin B12 is also essential for DNA synthesis, production of energy from fat and protein, and plays a key role in blood cell production. Sounds fancy, but it is a relatively cheap supplement. I usually get it about three months' worth at places like Whole Foods, Sprouts, Vitamin Shoppe, for roughly $8. Just be sure to look for the versions that are labeled "veg/vegan" because many forms of B12 are derived from animals.

Vitamin D

Another vitamin of extreme importance is Vitamin D. The common assumption about Vitamin D and veganism is that the two are not compatible. Which is bullshit.

If you walk down the cereal aisle or juice case in your local grocery store you will see a ton of products that are enriched with Vitamin D (most of which are not vegan, as the main dietary sources for most Vitamin D products are lanolin from sheep's wool or fish oil). But most people are not vegan (yet), not by a long shot, so why the hell do all these companies try to promote their products through the implication that their buyers need more Vitamin D?

That's because the natural way to get Vitamin D is not dietary. Rather, it is from sunlight, and the chemical reactions regulated by your skin to absorb sunlight and use it to strengthen your bones. The issue for most people, vegans and non-vegans alike, is that we simply don't get outside enough anymore. We sit at desks in front of computers more and more during our workdays. If we workout after work, we tend to workout indoors. We spend hours after work on Netflix or watching TV, and then we try to go to bed. And through all of this we miss out on the most essential source of vitality there ever was on Planet Earth: the light of the sun.

So before I send you into the health food store to buy a ten dollar bottle of vegan Vitamin D pills, perhaps consider trying to be more active in the sunlight more often. It's proven to give you more energy in your days as well as help you naturally produce more melatonin to rest easy at night.

However, supplementing with Vitamin D can still be helpful, and I would argue that it is essential, because as is the case with most people who don't live in the desert or near the beach, you're still likely not going to be exposed to enough direct sunlight to meet your Vitamin D needs on a daily basis. And like B12, vegan Vitamin D pills or liquids can be very cheap, and last you months on end for less than $20.

Two other solid Vitamin D options that I incorporate into my own diet at least some of the time are: eating UV-treated mushrooms, and/or getting a green superfood powder (like the Green Vibrance Daily Superfood product that I recommend in my meal plan—it not only has vegan D3 in it, but also vegan probiotics and a ton of essential vitamins and nutrients, too).

You need Vitamin D to maintain strong bones, and without strong bones there is no way to achieve Vegan Power. Therefore, I don't just recommend one solution to get your Vitamin D fix—I recommend all of the ones I listed here. Get out in the sun as much as you can. Take a Vitamin D supplement or use a green superfood powder that is specifically formulated to provide RDI of Vitamin D (like the one listed in my meal plan) in smoothies or shakes that has substantial Vitamin D quantities in it, and if you enjoy them enough—eat UV-treated mushrooms that you can likely find in just about any supermarket now. You will know they are the right ones because they will boast on the wrapper that they are an excellent source of Vitamin D.

Creatine

Do you want to be a Vegan Beast? If you read this far then I assume the answer is yes. Okay then, you don't have a choice but to supplement with creatine. Why? Because creatine is typically not found in plant-based foods. The good news is that most creatine on the market now is technically vegan because it is synthesized in laboratory environments.

Creatine is a compound of nitrogenous acid that muscles and brain tissue use as a fuel source. It is naturally found in the body, but usually at levels which won't meet the demands of someone trying to become a Vegan Beast, or a beast of any sorts. Creatine has many well-known benefits for lifters, or even just average civilians. It can help increase muscle fiber size, decrease muscle fatigue, improve muscle contraction, improve both maximal strength performance and repetitive endurance, improve cognitive function, and bone regeneration, among other things. Basically, creatine is fucking badass. It is especially noted for helping to improve muscle mass and performance for vegans and vegetarians due to vegans and vegetarians getting next to no creatine naturally through diet.

Another great thing about creatine is that it is cheap. I typically get several months' worth of creatine monohydrate powder (the most simple, trusted, and widely available form of creatine on the market) for less than $30, either at stores like Vitamin Shoppe or GNC, or for even cheaper via ordering on the True Nutrition website.

Creatine monohydrate is often said to upset the stomach, cause abdominal bloating, or gassiness. In my experience those claims can all be true to varying degrees, especially when you first begin taking creatine on a daily basis, but I have taken it nearly every day since late 2010, and for years now I can't recall noticing any of the symptoms listed above. Like with most things, your body will adapt to the changes you throw at it if you stay regular with new habits and substances. When I first started taking creatine I was generally only taking 5g a day in my protein shake right after my workouts. I recalled some bloating and gas back then, but I also noticed my muscles looking more full, or having a more pronounced "pump" from my workouts, so I promptly disregarded whatever physical discomfort I may have felt. It was nice to see that supplementation was yielding noticeable results, at least visually, almost immediately (within the same week I started using it).

Typical dosage for creatine is about 5g daily for the average person (a.k.a an omnivore), but due to it being a tricky compound for your body to absorb, it is possible that 80% or more of that dosage may not be absorbed when ingested. Like I said, I started taking 5g once daily more than six years ago. I was advised by another vegan lifter to not cycle on or off creatine like many bodybuilders do (meat-eaters especially) since there is virtually no creatine found in plant-based foods. It is true that it is possible, though not highly likely, that meat-eaters can get adequate levels of creatine from their "food" choices alone, but even so the body will not absorb much of it, and therefore omnivores still usually supplement with it, though with perhaps less than vegans may need to. I found over the years that as my stomach's tolerance for creatine increased (i.e. I had less bloating or gas) I could ramp up my dosage, so for a long while I took 10g a day. In 2015 though, for insurance purposes, I got a blood test done to check various levels of nutrients, minerals, and acids in my blood. My creatine levels showed to be within a healthy range but on the lower half of the healthy range, so I said "fuck it, time to start taking more creatine!" I currently take 15g of creatine monohydrate on a daily basis (5g with my morning smoothie, 5g with each shake or smoothie later on), and I never cycle off. Bloating is no issue. Gas is no issue. My blood work looks great. My urine and kidney function seem perfectly healthy. I can assuredly say that those discomforts of gas and bloating

I mentioned are likely initial, and that if you stick with a steady dosage you can improve your digestive tolerance for creatine, and likewise you will be able to increase your performance along the way.

There have been various times, when touring with my band especially, in which I have lapsed in taking creatine regularly, and then when I come home and get back in the gym, I notice I am considerably weaker than before the tour. It has happened to me enough times for me to believe that isn't a coincidence or just in my head. Creatine can make that big of a difference for you in just a matter of weeks. Now, when I travel, I keep creatine on hand and take it as regularly as I do when I am at home, in the gym or not.

Another common criticism of creatine is that it causes muscles to retain water, which in turn causes you to retain water weight, and therefore it makes you look "soft." If you care about strength, disregard these criticisms, as getting more water and fuel to your muscles with the help of creatine is going to help you increase muscle mass and strength overall because that is going to help you move more weight, and what else could you really want? I can attest that I have been able to gain muscle and strength without gaining weight for years now, and like I said, I do not cycle off creatine. It is very possible to take even a "high" dosage per day (like I do) and still not gain weight as you improve performance. You simply need to test your own tolerance for digesting creatine, as well as test what kind of results it gives you.

Overall though, just know this: creatine is badass, and if you want to be a Vegan Beast, you absolutely must take it on a daily basis.

OPTIONAL SUPPLEMENTS

L-Glutamine

Like creatine, glutamine (L-glutamine if you want to be specific) can go along way in helping you with recovery. Glutamine is the most abundant amino acid in the body, making up over 60% of skeletal muscle, but it really seems you can't have enough of it because it is the leading carrier of nitrogen in your body, and it can even boost metabolism and production of growth hormones (GAINS!). So it's kinda important. That goes for athletes of any kind, vegans and non-vegans alike.

I've been using glutamine for quite a few years now, maybe not quite as long as creatine, but definitely ever since I got ambitious about lifting. On average these days I take about 15g a day (5g per shake or smoothie, just as I do with creatine). I've experienced no side effects from glutamine consumption, and in general there are little to no known side effects in case studies. It's even a little cheaper than creatine, usually costing me $23-25 for a few months' worth of tasteless powder. If you want to be a Vegan Beast you need glutamine supplementation because it is crucial for helping advance recovery. That's really all there is to it.

Glucosamine

Though glucosamine also occurs naturally in the body, and is mostly associated with the protective fluid around your joints, it cannot be denied that if you are athlete who toils at your craft long enough and hard enough, you're very likely to inflame your tendons or experience some kind of joint pain at some point, whether you're lifting or just doing dreaded cardio (not sure why you'd do that, but whatever). Putting extra glucosamine in your body, alongside good stretching/self-myofascial release practices and adequate recovery time, can noticeably protect you from joint inflammation.

Finding vegan glucosamine can be tricky, because there are some brands out there who offer "vegetarian" glucosamine that has no gelatin, yet still uses shellfish sources for the actual glucosamine, and that shit just ain't going to cut it. Vegan glucosamine is derived from corn, and I find the best brand to get is DEVA brand, because they are an all-vegan company. But even ordering from them may be difficult, as they generally just sell to distributors, so I usually order their products online (just search on Google, ya know?). Whole Foods actually offers a vegan glucosamine, but I notice that not all Whole Foods stores tend to have it. It can be very hit or miss. Whatever you do though, don't get duped into buying non-vegan glucosamine. It may take some effort to get the vegan stuff, but if you live by your principles, you simply do what it takes, right? Right.

In 2015 I started to experience some knee pain, and it turned out to be patellar tendinitis. You would assume that I inflamed my knee from squatting like a madman for than five years straight, but really what happened was that I played a show with my band in Brooklyn one night, jumping around on stage like I do, then lugged my luggage from a friend's house the next morning up and down the streets and subways of NYC to go do a fucking *leg day* at a friend's gym in Manhattan, then lugged all my stuff back up to Red Bamboo in Washington Square to get fucked up on food, and then hoisted all my luggage some more straight to the airport. I remember sitting down at my gate at the airport that afternoon. I got up soon after to get some water, and it was precisely then that my left knee didn't feel right. All the stress over the previous twenty-four hours, with all its various strains and pressures on my knees, caught up with me. So many injuries come not from the stress we put on our bodies in the gym, but from the stress we put on our bodies outside of the gym *on top of* the stress we induced in the gym. And such was the case for me.

I had never taken glucosamine before because I had never experienced joint pain from lifting before, but I soon found I couldn't squat deep without severe pain in my left knee, so I had to go to a sports medicine doctor to get it checked out. From then on I began taking glucosamine regularly, as well as foam-rolling my legs regularly after workouts, and I have been squatting stronger than ever since my recovery from that case of tendinitis.

As is the case with any of the supplements I am talking about in this book, clear proof that they are giving us an edge in recovery or competition is certainly debatable and hard to quantify for anyone not participating in research about them, but I personally insist on taking these supplements because it is scientifically proven that the regular quantities of these substances that are either synthesized naturally in the body, or found naturally in food, are often not enough to compensate for the innumerable pressures and tensions strength training causes to the body, especially muscles, joints, and tendons. Strength athletes simply need more than the normal person eats or naturally creates in their body through natural process. As long as I am making incremental gains, it's all the comfort and proof I need, placebo or not. And plus, I figure it's better to be safe than sorry, even if it costs some money.

Calcium-Magnesium-Zinc

These are all minerals that you can get easily eating plant-based foods, and even on my meal plan you ought to get plenty of them through green vegetables, soy foods, nuts or nut butters, or even giving your veggies a little zing with some nutritional yeast now and then. However, like I have been saying, when you start lifting heavy, especially after you have been lifting heavy for years, your muscles need a little extra mineral boost. Magnesium and Zinc especially play a role in healthy muscle function, and Calcium is key for bone health and metabolism, so there is no way around supplementing these minerals, especially when your body starts to give you signals that you've been pushing yourself too hard for too long.

For example, a couple years ago I was laying in bed one night and my shoulder muscles, and sometimes my pec muscles, just started twitching. It didn't hurt or anything, but I'd be laying there perfectly still, and I'd have these weird twitches going on, and it started to make me think uncomfortable thoughts. So I started searching for the source of muscle twitches and spasms on the internet, and I commonly found that Magnesium deficiency was a common culprit for these kinds of symptoms, so I thought "Okay, I'll just get a Magnesium supplement, and see how it goes." And lucky for me, that seems to have done the trick. At that point I'd been into heavy lifting for more than four years, and never experienced twitching like that, but one point I like to make often in this book is that if you are ambitious about becoming strong, the stress on your body will almost definitely catch up with you in time. We all have our natural limits, and becoming stronger often means pushing yourself past those natural limits, and side effects are just part of collateral damage of your ambitions. So shrug your shoulders, say fuck it, and take your goddamn supplements to minimize the risk of injury or burnout, because when your body gives you little nudges (like muscle twitches when you are resting) that you need more of a certain something, you better listen and answer the call, or else there will be a more painful and expensive price to pay down the line. And even worse, you'll likely stop making gains.

Some of you may be thinking, "But Mr. Vegan Meathead, if you need all these supplements, your vegan diet must really be insufficient after all."

No, fuck you. Magnesium defciency, particularly, is so common that it is speculated that up to 80% of Americans experience it. I guarantee you that if you ate magnesium rich foods all the time, like I do (soy, beans, greens, bananas, nuts, sweet potatoes, even coffee) there is no reason someone who isn't ambitiously athletic should get enough mineral-intake to meet their daily needs. But just look at any competitive bodybuilder who isn't vegan. You think those maniacs got to be that big and jacked with less than what I am proposing you utilize in this book? L-O-fucking-L. What I am promoting in this book is very minimal supplementation compared to the supplemental circus that those vein-popping maniacs on magazine covers are taking, I promise you. Let's not even talk about steroids. Good lord…

As for Zinc, it must be replenished daily. It is found in a lot of the same foods as Magnesium and Calcium, but your body does not absorb it or store it as well. Fortunately, you'll often find it in the very same supplement formulas or pills that have Magnesium and Calcium, the trifecta of bone and muscle health. See, simple solutions for vegan strength and health, as always.

Pre-Workout Formulas

I'm a little on the fence about pre-workout formulas. After years of trying a few, I have decided that in some ways I think they provide a placebo effect more than anything. Most pre-workout formulas are predominantly a mix of Glutamine, Creatine, Arginine, and Beta-Alanine, perhaps with Caffeine or Taurine as well. There is plenty of evidence to back up that these amino acids or substances can reliably increase your performance by a smidge. And a little smidge consistently over time adds up to perhaps between the difference between good and great conditioning, but at the same time it is true that sometimes you really can't tell if these substances are helping. Perhaps they help simply because they give you a little tingle and you want them to help you.

One argument that I have heard against using pre-workout supplements is that they will gradually desensitize your adrenal glands, and what happens then is that you need more and more of whatever powdered formula to keep amping you up, and it just never seems to end. For example, you'll start out using one-and-a-half scoops of some fruit punch flavored powder thirty minutes before you hit the gym, but a year later you need three-and-a-half to get the same feeling.

Likewise, I have gotten all buzzed up from the Beta-Alanine tingle, for years of my workout history, but there have been plenty of times I have still gotten in the squat rack or on the bench and missed my lifts all the same. Not only that, but pre-workout formulas aren't exactly cheap. A lot of times they will run you $30-40 a month, if not more, and for me personally I don't know if it is worth it anymore, especially as I have come to need more and more servings to get me buzzing and amped up to lift.

So just know, there are some decent vegan (or technically vegan) options out there for pre-workout formulas, or for the amino acids I listed above, but it is also fair to say you may not need them. Maybe give them a try? It's really up to you.

At this point, what I like to do is have a cup of coffee, put a half-serving of creatine in it, and maybe add a half teaspoon of coconut oil for quick energy. I can't really say for sure that the caffeine gives my system a jolt anymore, but the truth is that the ritual is nice. It gets me in the mindset of saying "Alright dude, it's about to be Hero Time! Time to go crush some weight!" Plus, I really love drinking coffee.

More than anything, my point here is that I don't think there is any certain way to know how much a pre-workout substance or formula is going to help you excel in your workouts, so just opt for doing or consuming something that makes you believe you are destined to go make some serious progress with the weights, something that helps you tell yourself that it is indeed "Hero Time." Time to shine.

THINGS TO NOT WORRY ABOUT

Don't worry about Iron. If you follow my meal plan, you'll see that you get more than enough Iron. Women do need to consume more iron than men, so that is something to consider, but my meal plan provides ample iron.

Don't worry about Vitamin C. If you eat green vegetables every day and some fruit, like in my meal plan, you will get plenty of Vitamin C.

Don't worry about fiber. I am actually trying to reduce your fiber intake through my meal plan so you can increase potential time in the gut absorb minerals, nutrients, and micronutrients. Being vegan alone is nearly a fail-safe for getting more than enough fiber. Can you believe that we live in a time and place where people (and by "people" I mean *adult* omnivores) actually buy gummy bear candy vitamins to supplement fiber? Holy fuck, America, you are doomed.

Don't worry about amino acids in general, because if you are supplementing with a good protein powder and eating the variety of foods in my meal plan, guess what? You're more than fucking covered.

Alright, at last, the moment you've been waiting for…

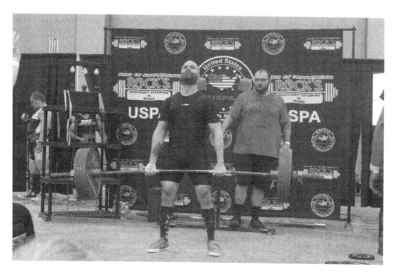
A triple bodyweight deadlift. JK, on to the meal plan...
(Photo: Robert Cheeke)

THE VEGAN MEATHEAD MEAL PLAN

BEFORE WE GET DOWN to business here, and I show you the specific numbers of calories, servings, times, and items I eat on a regular basis, keep some things in mind:

1) This is a meal plan for a roughly 165 pound male who does compound lifts at a minimum of three days a week, usually. Sometimes more, sometimes less depending on all kinds of factors. For powerlifters, like myself, it is speculated that the ideal bodyfat range is 8-15%. Too little fat is known to hamper testosterone production, which reduces your ability to build muscle, just as too much fat will do the same. On this diet I have steadily held around 10-13% for years now, primarily by lifting regularly and eating as close to this schedule as possible.

2) I cannot guarantee this will work for you as well as me, but it was generally adapted from a bodybuilding meal plan, tweaked to accommodate my personal needs, which did not include such an extreme need for fat loss as that which a bodybuilder typically requires to get "shredded." Bodybuilders ideally compete with their body compositions in the 3-7% range of bodyfat, and in my experience, trying to get that low is just plain painful.

3) I do not support the "bulking" and "cutting" methods of dieting that bodybuilders typically implement, because I am not a bodybuilder, and there are even bodybuilders who see the futility of bulking and cutting cycles as well. I instead advocate for slow gains that require no period of weight loss, because I do not see the point of building a bunch of strength while accumulating more bodyweight that you cannot keep for competition. When people "cut" after a diligent bulking period, they often lose a lot of their strength and size with the weight they in turn shed to get more defined. While maintaining body fat within the 8-15% range recommended for peak strength performance, looking "cut" or exceptionally defined is irrelevant. It also an illusion of strength much of the time, as bodybuilders often make their muscles pop out and look bigger, even though they can typically move less weight. Besides, at that range of bodyfat (8-15%), you are going to look solid as fuck, and you will be solid as fuck. Maybe you can get "cut" on an eating plan like this while lifting for strength, as some people naturally will become so easier than others, but it is not the goal. This meal plan is meant to give you a roadmap to make incremental gains that you won't lose.

4) By all means, feel free to play around with the calorie math to be in accord with your current body mass. For example, if you're a 300-pound football player who wants to succeed on a vegan diet, you'll simply have to eat two Tofurky sausages instead of one. It's expensive being a big guy, I know, but obeying the mathematical demands of your metabolism is imperative. The bigger you are the more calories and protein you need to consume. And likewise, if you're a woman who perhaps weighs 115-125 pounds, let's say for example, then you only need to eat roughly 75% of the portions I am listing here.

5) As you are about to see, this is an obscene amount of protein, even for an omnivore. I figure it's best to overshoot than to fall short. When someone can produce a relevant study or series of studies that indisputably show the detrimental effects of plant protein when consumed in excess, maybe then I will reconsider. But until then, this is how I party. So far so good for me.

LIFTING DAY MEAL PLAN

7:00 AM - Breakfast

Beyond Meat Grilled Chicken Strips (approx. 9 strips)
180 calories, 30g protein, 9g carb, 4.5g fat, 3g fiber, 30% RDV iron, 0g sugar

Coconut Oil (1 Tbsp, used for grilling in pan)
120 calories, 14g fat, no protein, carb, fiber, iron, sugar

Annie's Goddess Dressing (2 Tbsp, for dipping)

120 calories, 1g protein, 2g carb, 12g fat, no fiber, iron, sugar

Coffee (1 Cup, black)
Soy Creamer (1 Tbsp, optional)

20 calories, 2g carb, 1.5g fat, 1g sugar

Breakfast TOTAL: 440 calories, 31g protein, 13g carb, 32g fat, 3g fiber, 30% RDV Iron, 1g sugar

****

9:30 AM - Smoothie
Water (filtered, 20 oz.)

NitroFusion chocolate protein powder (1 scoop, 30g)

120 calories, 21g protein, 4g carb, 2g fat, 4g sugar, no fiber, no Iron

Mixed Berries (frozen, 1/2 cup)

40 calories, 1g protein, 7.5g carb, .5g fat, 3g fiber, 4% RDV Iron, 2.5g sugar

Green Vibrance Daily Superfood Powder (1 scoop, 11.83g)

40 calories, 2g protein, 1g carb, .5g fiber, 2g fiber, 20% RDV Iron, 1g sugar

L-Glutamine Powder (1 scoop, 4.5g)

no significant macronutrient values

Creatine Monohydrate Powder (1 scoop, 5g)

no significant macronutrient values

Peanut Butter (optional if lifting heavy that day, 1.5 Tbsp)

147 calories, 5g protein, 4.5g carb, 12g fat, 2.5g fiber, 4.5% RDV Iron, 1g sugar

Tofu (extra firm, 1/4 block)

90 calories, 10g protein, 3.5g carb, 4.5g fat, 1g fiber, 9% RDV Iron, no sugar

*Blend all of this together (obviously)

Smoothie TOTAL: 437 calories, 39g protein, 20.5g carb, 19.5g fat, 8.5g fiber, 37.5% RDV Iron, 8.5g sugar

****

12:00 PM - Lunch #1

Tofurky Italian Sausage (1 link)

280 calories, 30g protein, 8g carb, 14g fat, 1g fiber, 20% RDV Iron, 3g sugar

Broccoli (1 cup, frozen or fresh, steamed or cooked)

15 calories, 1g protein, 3 carb, .25g fat, 1g fiber, 1% RDV Iron, .75 sugar

Lunch #1 TOTAL: 295 calories, 31g protein, 11g carb, 14.25g fat, 2g fiber, 21% RDV Iron, 3.75 sugar

****

2:30 PM - Protein Shake

Water (filtered, 16 oz.)

Nitro Fusion chocolate protein powder **(1 scoop, 30g)**

120 calories, 21g protein, 4g carb, 2g fat, 4g sugar, no fiber, no Iron

L-Glutamine Powder (1 scoop, 4.5g)

no significant macronutrient values

Creatine Monohydrate Powder (1 scoop, 5g)

no significant macronutrient values

Protein Shake TOTAL: 120 calories, 21g protein, 4g carb, 2g fat, 4g fiber, no sugar, no Iron

****

4:30 PM - Lunch #2

Tofurky Italian Sausage (1 link)

280 calories, 30g protein, 8g carb, 14g fat, 1g fiber, 20% RDV Iron, 3g sugar

Broccoli or Cauliflower (1 cup, frozen or fresh, steamed or cooked)

15 calories, 1g protein, 3 carb, .25g fat, 1g fiber, 1% RDV Iron, .75 sugar

Lunch #1 TOTAL: 295 calories, 31g protein, 11g carb, 14.25g fat, 2g fiber, 21% RDV Iron, 3.75 sugar

****

6:30 PM - Pre-Workout Snack

Clif Builder Bar (1 bar)

280 calories, 20g protein, 29 carb, 10g fat, 2g fiber, 15% RDV Iron, 21g sugar

Coffee (1 Cup, black)
Soy Creamer (1 Tbsp, optional)

20 calories, 2g carb, 1.5g fat, 1g sugar

Pre-Workout Snack TOTAL: 300 calories, 20g protein, 31g carb, 11.5g fat, 2g fiber, 15% RDV Iron, 22g sugar

8-8:30 PM - Post-Workout Protein and Carb Load

Lenny & Larry's Complete Cookie (1 whole cookie)

400 calories, 16g protein, 54g carb, 12g fat, 8g fiber, 22% RDV Iron, 30g sugar

Daiya Dairy-Free Greek Yogurt or Silk Dairy-Free Yogurt (1 cup)

150 calories, 8g protein, 20g carb, 4.5g fat, 3g fiber, 10% RDV Iron, 13g sugar

Smoothie
Water (filtered, 20 oz.)

NitroFusion chocolate protein powder (1 scoop, 30g)

120 calories, 21g protein, 4g carb, 2g fat, 4g sugar, no fiber, no Iron

Banana (frozen, 1/2 piece)

50 calories, .5g protein, 13.5g carb, .25g fat, 1.5g fiber, .50% RDV Iron, 7g sugar

L-Glutamine Powder (1 scoop, 4.5g)

no significant macronutrient values

Creatine Monohydrate Powder (1 scoop, 5g)

no significant macronutrient values

Raw Spinach or Kale (1 handful)

10 calories, .5g protein, .5g carb, .5g fiber, 2% RDV Iron, no fat, no sugar

Tofu (extra firm, 1/4 block)

90 calories, 10g protein, 3.5g carb, 4.5g fat, 1g fiber, 9% RDV Iron, 0g sugar

*Blend all of this together (obviously)

Post-Workout TOTAL: 820 calories, 56g protein, 95.5g carb, 23.25g fat, 14g fiber, 43.5% RDV Iron, 54g sugar

10:30 PM - Bedtime Snack

Tofurky Deli Slices (5 plain slices)

100 calories, 13g protein, 6g carb, 3g fat, 3g fiber, 6% RDV Iron, 1g sugar

****

Lifting Day COMPLETE TOTAL:

2807 calories
242g protein
192g carb
119.75g fat
34.5g fiber
174% RDV Iron
98g sugar

Macronutrient Calorie Percentages:

Protein = 34.5%
Carbohydrate = 27.25%
Fat = 38.25%

Notes:

Always experiment with your own tolerance for creatine monohydrate. I consume 5g three times a day because my bloodwork has shown I can handle it and keep within a healthy range. I also have conditioned myself to not be bloated or have upset stomach from creatine, yet many people who try to consume it struggle with those kinds of issues. When I first started incorporating creatine into my diet in 2010, I definitely got bloated and gassy, and back then I started with only one 5g serving in my shake per day. Later I graduated to two per day, and recently to three. If you are expecting to build muscle and strength on a vegan diet, I recommend using creatine despite the initial discomfort it causes for many people.

Creatine is not naturally found in most plant-based foods, at least not in significant quantities, so there is also no need to "cycle on" or off of it as omnivores do. I have consumed creatine powder nearly everyday for the past 7 years, have shown to have healthy bloodwork, kidney function and urine analysis. As always, you should be drinking plenty of water with and in between meals, especially on a high protein diet like this one.

I also sometimes sub Annie's Goddess Dressing in the morning for Chipotle Vegenaise or Just Mayo. Both are high fat like Goddess Dressing, and taste great too. The purpose of using either of these is to get your fat consumption up first thing in the day. All 3 do the trick.

You can also sub half an avocado or almond butter for peanut butter in the smoothie.

Regarding the cooked or steamed vegetables you eat at various times of the day, do not cook them in oil. There are already enough fat calories in this diet. Cook or steam your vegetables in a splash of water in a pot if you are at home and able. When I used to eat my lunches at a shared office space, I would save frozen greens in the company fridge, then 'steam' a serving of them in a microwave with by creating a makeshift pressure cooker with either two bowls or a plate over a bowl to trap the heat and moisture in. It usually wouldn't take more than two minutes in the microwave to get the veggies ready that way. It wasn't fancy by any means, but it sure beat meal-prepping.

REGULAR OFF DAY / MAINTENANCE MEAL PLAN

7:00 AM - Breakfast

Beyond Meat Grilled Chicken Strips (approx. 9 strips)
180 calories, 30g protein, 9g carb, 4.5g fat, 3g fiber, 30% RDV iron, 0g sugar

Coconut Oil (1 Tbsp, used for grilling in pan)
120 calories, 14g fat, no protein, carb, fiber, iron, sugar

Annie's Goddess Dressing (2 Tbsp, for dipping)
120 calories, 1g protein, 2g carb, 12g fat, no fiber, iron, sugar

Coffee (1 Cup, black)
Soy Creamer (1 Tbsp, optional)
20 calories, 2g carb, 1.5g fat, 1g sugar

Breakfast TOTAL: 440 calories, 31g protein, 13g carb, 32g fat, 3g fiber, 30% RDV Iron, 1g sugar

****

9:30 AM - Smoothie

Water (filtered, 20 oz.)

NitroFusion chocolate protein powder (1 scoop, 30g)
120 calories, 21g protein, 4g carb, 2g fat, 4g sugar, no fiber, no Iron

Mixed Berries (frozen, 1/2 cup)
40 calories, 1g protein, 7.5g carb, .5g fat, 3g fiber, 4% RDV Iron, 2.5g sugar

Green Vibrance Daily Superfood Powder (1 scoop, 11.83g)

40 calories, 2g protein, 1g carb, .5g fiber, 2g fiber, 20% RDV Iron, 1g sugar

L-Glutamine Powder (1 scoop, 4.5g)

no significant macronutrient values

Creatine Monohydrate Powder (1 scoop, 5g)

no significant macronutrient values

Tofu (extra firm, 1/4 block)

90 calories, 10g protein,/ 3.5g carb, 4.5g fat, 1g fiber, 9% RDV Iron, no sugar

*Blend all of this together (obviously)

Smoothie TOTAL: 290 calories, 34g protein, 16g carb, 7.5g fat, 6g fiber, 30% RDV Iron, 1g sugar

****

12:00 PM - Lunch #1

Beyond Meat Beefy Crumbles (1/3 bag)

200 calories, 26g protein, 6g carb, 10g fat, 4g fiber, 4% RDV Iron, 2g sugar

Broccoli (1 cup, frozen or fresh, steamed or cooked)

15 calories, 1g protein, 3 carb, .25g fat, 1g fiber, 1% RDV Iron, .75 sugar

Lunch #1 TOTAL: 215 calories, 27g protein, 9g carb, 10.25g fat, 5g fiber, 5% RDV Iron, 2.75 sugar

2:30 PM - Protein Shake

Water (filtered, 16 oz.)

Nitro Fusion chocolate protein powder (1 scoop, 30g)
120 calories, 21g protein, 4g carb, 2g fat, 4g sugar, no fiber, no Iron

L-Glutamine Powder (1 scoop, 4.5g)
no significant macronutrient values

Creatine Monohydrate Powder (1 scoop, 5g)
no significant macronutrient values

Protein Shake TOTAL: 120 calories, 21g protein, 4g carb, 2g fat, 4g fiber, no sugar, no Iron

****

4:30 PM - Lunch #2

Beyond Meat Beefy Crumbles (1/3 bag)
200 calories, 26g protein, 6g carb, 10g fat, 4g fiber, 4% RDV Iron, 2g sugar

Greens (1 cup, frozen or fresh, steamed or cooked)
15 calories, 1g protein, 3 carb, .25g fat, 1g fiber, 1% RDV Iron, .75 sugar

Lunch #1 TOTAL: 215 calories, 27g protein, 9g carb, 10.25g fat, 5g fiber, 5% RDV Iron, 2.75 sugar

****

6:30 PM - Snack

NuGo Slim Chocolate Peanut Butter Bar (1 bar)
180 calories, 17g protein, 19 carb, 7g fat, 7g fiber, 8% RDV Iron, 2g sugar

Coffee (1 Cup, black)
Soy Creamer (1 Tbsp, optional)

20 calories, 2g carb, 1.5g fat, 1g sugar

Snack TOTAL: 200 calories, 17g protein, 21g carb, 8.5g fat, 7g fiber, 8% RDV Iron, 3g sugar

****

8:00 PM - Dinner

Gardein Sweet and Sour Porkless Bites (1 full package, use 1/2 packet of sauce only)

410 calories, 39g protein, 39g carb, 9g fat, 6g fiber, 30% RDV Iron, 15g sugar

Kale (2 cups, sauteed with garlic, turmeric, soy sauce)

65 calories, 6g protein, 12g carb, 1g fat, 2g fiber, 10% RDV Iron, no sugar

Dinner TOTAL: 475 calories, 45g protein, 51g carb, 10g fat, 8g fiber, 40% RDV Iron, 15g sugar

****

10:30 PM - Protein Shake and Bedtime Snack

Water (filtered, 16 oz.)

Nitro Fusion chocolate protein powder **(1 scoop, 30g)**

120 calories, 21g protein, 4g carb, 2g fat, 4g sugar, no fiber, no Iron

L-Glutamine Powder (1 scoop, 4.5g)

no significant macronutrient values

Creatine Monohydrate Powder (1 scoop, 5g)

no significant macronutrient values

Snack

Daiya Dairy-Free Greek Yogurt or Silk Dairy-Free Yogurt (1 cup)

150 calories, 8g protein, 20g carb, 4.5g fat, 3g fiber, 10% RDV Iron, 13g sugar

Shake and Snack TOTAL: 270 calories, 29g protein, 24g carb, 6.5g fat, 3g fiber, 10% RDV Iron, 17g sugar

****

Off Day / Maintenance COMPLETE TOTAL:

2225 calories
231g protein
147g carb
87g fat
37g fiber
131% RDV Iron
49g sugar

Macronutrient Calorie Percentages:

Protein = 41.5%
Carbohydrate = 26.5%
Fat = 32%

More Notes:

I do not necessarily eat this exact way on every off-day from lifting, but it is pretty close, and on many off-days I DO eat precisely this.

A good substitute for the Gardein Porkless Bites are just about any other Gardein dinner, like the Beefless Tips, Teriyaki Chicken or Meatless Meatloaf.

Again, cook your vegetables in water. Do not add oil!

SOME THOUGHTS ABOUT TRAINING

I DECIDED to forego giving training advice in this book, simply because what works for each one of us is often too individualized and specific to our state of health, fitness conditioning, and desired goals for me to give one-size-fits-all suggestions on what kind of workouts you should be doing. In contrast, the principles of eating that I have outlined in this book give you concrete quantities to work with and adapt based on your metabolism, body mass, nutritional demands to meet training goals, and whatever other self-knowledge you attain in your fitness development that may require you to play with the numbers to keep meeting your goals. You'll always find that you have to adjust numbers as you go along, in diet and training alike, based on whatever circumstances you find yourself in. Hopefully the information I have presented to you helps you navigate your own path with a basis of useful reference in regards to eating for strength.

As I have said many times throughout this book, my way of eating is primarily meant to accommodate strength athletes, but I wholeheartedly think this kind of diet could be utilized by crossfitters, kettlebellers, and other kinds of athletes who mix strength with endurance. However, the more one's fitness goals are based on endurance, the less I would recommend following The Way of The Vegan Meathead. Nevertheless, if you want to put on mass and build strength to any degree, I think my meal plan can be of great use to you, whether you are a beginning lifter, intermediate, or advanced. You can be running a 5x5 powerlifting/bodybuilding program, doing high rep definition work, circuit training, high intensity powerlifting or strongman type routines, and the quantities and proportions of fat, protein, and carbs I am proposing you abide by should be sufficient to help you make the gains you seek, as they have been for me.

I started eating this way in late 2014, and at that time I weighed nearly 180 pounds, but was lucky to clear 1000 pounds on my big 3 lifts. Once I started eating like this I began to whittle away the weight, and I competed in my first powerlifting meet in June 2015, weighing in at 161 pounds and putting up a 1045 total. A year later, at the same meet I had gained no weight and put up an 1146 total, a Class 1 total in the United States Powerlifting Association (USPA), which means I can qualify to compete in national level competitions. As I write this I am still maintaining weight under 165 pounds, and I am just shy of a 1200 pound total.

As I said some chapters ago, I am an advocate of the slow and sustainable gains. This diet has allowed me just that, but I assure you I have varied my training up constantly between the time I started eating this way and now.

Another reason I cannot in good conscience talk about training in this book is that each us of have unique frames and genetic builds that give us greater aptitude in certain types of sports than others. It's really up to you to figure what you like most and what you're best at, and then go for it.

For example, before I got into powerlifting I was trying to more or less to be a bodybuilder, following bodybuilding type programs and diet schedules to build my physique. I found that I was gradually getting leaner looking, and while that was satisfying in some regard, I didn't like the fact that I wasn't getting much stronger, especially for all the work I was putting in. I found that I enjoy the progress of seeing my numbers go up on a chart more than getting a little more definition in my abs week by week. Plus, I just never seemed to have the body type that could get vivid ab definition without starving the fuck out of myself, which in turn made me weaker when handling weights, and that in itself made me feel deflated and unaccomplished. Every time I did a cutting cycle I was miserable. I spent hours doing cardio sometimes, and that was also boring and miserable to me. Again, I am not knocking the peoplewho enjoy that stuff or who it comes naturally to, but my point is that it wasn't a good fit for me, partially because my body just didn't ever seem to sync up with the goals I was after.

So I consulted with a good friend who had run a 5x5 powerlifting program a couple times and said he had undeniable success with it. He sent me a link with a spreadsheet template and said after running it twice with some time off in between each cycle his squat and deadlift were going through the roof. Assuredly, he was experiencing beginner gains (which are so much fun, aren't they? Like falling in love...), but I was intrigued to experience the kind of satisfaction he was feeling, because I simply was not getting it from doing bodybuilding split routines and tons of cardio week after week just so I could look a certain way that often felt unattainable or unsustainable.

When I first started concentrating on my big 3 lifts (squat, bench, deadlift) and ran my first 5x5 cycle, it required me to stop doing cardio. I soon noticed that I was using the calories I had previously burned up by doing regular cardio to grow my muscles and become much stronger. My numbers started going through the roof as well. And when I'd walk into work back then, co-workers started giving me that aesthetic recognition I'd been seeking when doing those split body-building routines. (Don't lie, motherfuckers, we're all after some kind of recognition. At the very least, we all indisputably like it when we get it.)

"Damn Daniel, you're getting swole!"

"Dude, are you eating meat? You're looking strong."

"Watch out! Here comes the gun show!"

Maybe I wasn't getting chiseled under my shirt, not to the extent bodybuilders aim to, but I was getting bigger and filling my shirts and jeans out, and people were taking notice. I was starting to feel like I was accomplishing something.

Once I got deeper into the powerlifting lifestyle, where your whole life starts to be based around your three or four serious lifting days a week, and all your meal-planning is done to accommodate those lifting days, I soon discovered that because I am short, I had somewhat of a gift for power-lifting, especially squatting and deadlifting, because being short means the barbell has to travel a shorter distance for you to complete the lift than if I was six-foot-something. For once in my life being short seemed to be an advantage (though there are plenty of gifted powerlifters who are tall as well). If nothing else, powerlifting was coming more naturally to me than getting ripped like a bodybuilder, and was more enjoyable than running, so in time I gave up any aspirations of looking like some lean underwear model or vein-popping hulk-demon. I started to solely take pride in my strength and putting more weight on the bar. I also soon realized by mingling with other dudes doing compound lifts in the gym that most often the strongest people around aren't the leanest looking ones. I'd found my calling and place in the fitness arena.

And this is why if you have training questions, you either need to do your own homework about what kinds of training are best for you, or seek professional consultation, or both. We're all going to be best at different things, and different types of training will benefit us differently, so there is no substitute for trial, error, experience, and professional counsel about your individual conditioning and potentials.

Furthermore, I can't suggest specific programming in this book for anyone because you'll find that as you go along on your path to becoming a Vegan Beast almost every kind of program you can run to get stronger will quit working for you. You'll be lucky if a program works twice for you. You will then have to do your research to find new ways to trick your body to get stronger and grow. I've run beginner 5x5 programs, intermediate 5x5 programs, Smolov high frequency programs, deadlift specialist programs, auto-regulating programs, other programs that employ periodization, and lately I've become so desperate to keep making progress that I quit doing specific programming in order to listen to what my body needs in terms of stimulation and recovery, because the longer you keep lifting heavy, the harder it becomes to exceed your natural limits (this is what is referred to as the *advanced* stage of conditioning, where you may toil for months to achieve just a smidge of the progress you made in weeks when you started lifting). In order to break those kinds of plateaus you have to incorporate new things in to your repertoire, and you'll potentially have to tweak your diet, too.

But I will say, overall, that diet seems to be more static than training methods. Diet is the base of all you do. It is how you fuel yourself and partially how you heal yourself. There will always be base caloric and nutrient needs to be met, and that will never drastically change unless you drastically change your training goals. There is a balance between training capacity and dietary demand that you will always have to figure out for yourself. I sincerely hope you experience the kind of success and productivity I have experienced eating this way for several years now.

GO FORTH NOW WITH A RIGHTEOUS MISSION

NOW YOU HAVE a template from which to work from. You have a basic understanding of the different ways your metabolism can operate if you switch up fat calories and carbs, or eat fat and carbs at specific and appropriate times of the day, as well as the importance of eating more protein on a regular basis. Hopefully you see how easy it is to eat a high protein vegan diet for strength. And of course, more than anything, I hope you take your motherfucking B12 on a daily basis. And if you can retain some pointers about other supplementation for achieving Vegan Power, that is excellent too.

This book has not been about telling you the one way to achieve plant-based strength. Assuredly, there are many ways, and likewise I cannot even guarantee that this will work for you based on all the different possible factors that may vary between us, like age, metabolism, and overall health and conditioning. This is just my way, and it has been working for me, consistently, so I stand by it. Achieving the balance of being able to maintain or gradually shed weight while also gradually increasing strength is a conundrum so many of us face or have faced that I am simply happy to share with you my successful experiences of eating for strength, gradual weight loss, and maintenance. Once it is broken down, I think anyone can see that this approach to eating for strength is so simple it *is* stupid. The meals aren't fancy. Tofurky sausage and broccoli? Beyond Meat Chicken and salad dressing? Come on, it doesn't get easier than that. The diet overall is not expensive, and it typically doesn't even require meal prepping. Yes, supplements and protein powders can add up monetarily, but if you want to be good at something, you have to invest in it. And more than anything it is an investment in yourself, as well as one for a better world.

Let's envision a world where there are no more excuses for eating animals, for enslaving them, or killing them, where they are free to live their own lives as they please, just as we wish for ourselves and those we hold dear. For each of us who leads by example and cultivates our own health and strength, we represent something much bigger than ourselves. Simultaneously, we can exemplify a way of life that not only benefits animals and the environment, but one that benefits ourselves every bit as much.

Veganism is no sacrifice. It can be a way to thrive and become a beast, and given the available options to all of us these days, it is less challenging to achieve Vegan Power than ever before. So eat to win, and prove how easy it is time and time again. Envision a culture where people see a juggernaut stepping up to a barbell, handling weight that bends it, and their initial reaction is consistently: "Damn, he/she must be vegan."

Be *that* vegan.

The momentum is building, and the rise of the vegan is already happening on cultural levels, as the interest of the public is perpetually piqued, so now it's time to blow the gates open. It's time to do your part, to overcome yourself and become a better and stronger self than you ever thought you were capable of—for yourself, the animals, and the future of our own species. Consider it a calling to greatness.

Let's see what you've got.

The way of compassion should not be tread lightly
The path of culture is set by the mighty
Go forth now with a righteous mission
And do not relent until its completion

Expose the myths of the omnivore for what they are
Go forth and make the world understand
The Age of The Meat-Eater
Will come to an end

(Band of Mercy)

ACKNOWLEDGEMENTS

I am grateful to my father, Kenrick Albaugh, and my stepmom, Annette Albaugh, both for their unwavering belief in my ability to carry out this project and articulate my message. My dad was vehemently unhappy about me deciding to give up meat in my teen years, but these days he sees how far I have come and jokes that he "wants to be like me when he grows up." It is great fortune to have proud and adoring parents. Thank you both.

My mother, Jamey Ray, has always been the rock in my life. 2017 was not an easy year for me on a personal level, but she was always there to help me stabilize myself, no matter how far apart we were, and ultimately having that stability was the foundation that allowed me to find my balance and get back to being productive. Also, being that she stopped eating meat long before I was born, I'd say she had more than just a little influence on developing the compassionate streak that led me to embrace veganism.

I owe a lot to the knowledge and expertise of Carly Slawson, R.D., who helped guide my delivery for many of the harder to explain nutritional concepts in this book. Nutritional science is complicated, often up for debate, and communicating these concepts can be very difficult for a lay-person like me. Working with Carly was a valuable learning experience, and her benevolent nature helped me round off some of the jagged edges that may have alienated more people in the audience than I had intended. Carly, I know you can't stand by all the statements I have made in this book on a nutritional science level, not entirely anyway (LOL), but your overall influence on this project has been profound.

Garrett Huls of Huls Design was a delight to work with. The response I've gotten to his logo design has been nothing but positive. He came highly recommended by friends who launched brands he designed for, and I can say his contributions have been invaluable to The Style of The Vegan Meathead.

Marc Strömberg graced this book with his artistic talent. I am lucky to have an artist contact me with such excitement about the project, and to capture perfectly the vibe I wanted for Vegan Meathead.Thank you, Marc! I wish you all the best with all your projects and hope to work with you more. RHINO RAGE!

I had some friends volunteer to read and unofficially edit this book. Sal Fuentes, mi hermano del diablo, is always a great creative partner and prime encourager in all my creative endeavors. Chris "Conflict" Hatfield (notably of Underdog Apparel), despite being a complete caveman stuck in the modern age, actually found a few typos—which means he actually read the damn thing with intense attention to detail. I am impressed, dude! Didn't know you had it in you.

I can't thank my mentors and peers in Vegan Power enough for their support of me and this book: my PlantBuilt family beginning with Jason Patton, Giacomo Marchese and Dani Taylor, Ed Bauer, Holly Noll, Natalie and George Matthews, the PlantBuilt powerlifters (Ndem, Paul, Jessica, Crystal, Lil Sara, and Anastasia), Forest Crosbie, Scott Shetler, and truly too many list here; the Letten brothers (Phil and Matt a.k.a. Vegan Bros.); my old friend, the ever-inspirational Toni Okamoto; Big Bald Mike Crockett (shout out to the dream of Bonebreaker Barbell!); Christy Morgan for her interest in seeing this project grow and *attempting* to share her social media prowess with me; and last but not least, Robert Cheeke, for inspiring me (and so many of us vegan athletes) on this path of health and compassion. Thumbs up!

I started writing this book in Summer of 2016, and I wrote more than half of it in a month or so, like magic that was meant to be, but then 2017 happened, and completing this project, as well as launching the Vegan Meathead brand, took a lot more concentration and diligence than I could have anticipated. I am deeply grateful to the folks out there who follow me online, whether close friends or not, who have found inspiration in my approach to promoting both veganism and a strength-based lifestyle, as well as simply caring to any degree about my own progress as a powerlifter. You may never know it, but your encouragement and excitement about The Vegan Meathead does help me keep my mind properly in the game, especially when I've most needed it, so thank you all. I wish you endless gains, and hope the content I offer may continue to be a valuable resource to you on your own path.

Through Vegan Power, all things are possible.

Daniel Austin
January 7, 2018

Made in the USA
Lexington, KY
13 November 2018